£4

GW00691671

THE ASTROLOGY OF ACCIDENTS

THE ASTROLOGY OF ACCIDENTS

Investigations and Research

By

CHARLES E. O. CARTER

Author of

An Encyclopædia of Psychological Astrology
The Principles of Astrology
The Seven Great Problems of Astrology
The Zodiac and the Soul
Symbolic Directions in Modern Astrology
The Astrological Aspects

THEOSOPHICAL PUBLISHING HOUSE LTD
68 Great Russell Street London WC1B 3BU

ADYAR-INDIA   WHEATON ILL.-USA

Reprinted 1977

SBN 7229 5059 4 (paperback)
SBN 7229 5045 4 (cased)

Printed in Great Britain by
Fletcher & Son Ltd, Norwich

CONTENTS

ACCURACY OF DATA

Where no reference is given, all nativities used or quoted herein are from private sources, and the time should be assumed to be as recorded. No cases are quoted unless I have reason to suppose that the time of birth is at least approximately accurate. It will be clear that it would be impossible to rectify a large number of maps, of which many are of persons whose lives, except as stated in this book, are unknown to me.

INTRODUCTION

THE present work is small in size, but it has involved a considerable amount of work during the years 1929, 1930, and 1931.

Modesty does not forbid me to claim for it the merit of being a valuable compilation of accident-horoscopes, for it is to others more than to me that the astrological world owes its thanks on this head. It would be invidious to mention many names in this connection, for assistance has come from several sources. However, I ought to mention with special gratitude the Swiss *savant*, K. E. Krafft, and George H. Bailey, of Bath, both of whom furnished a number of cases, whilst the first part of the book is really an echo—albeit a feeble one—of a series of lectures delivered to the Astrological Lodge some years ago by the former. Mr. Bailey also most kindly helped me with the rather arduous task of preparing this work for press.

The first part of the book is statistical, the results being arranged in three tables.

The statistical method has advantages, and, like most other things of which this may be said, also the defects of its virtues.

It is objective, stating, but not explaining, facts. It is unhampered by questions of the personal element, for the compiler is but an automaton, recording what he finds. It forms a most valuable commentary on traditional astrology, with which it sometimes agrees and sometimes disagrees, whilst at other times it amplifies what the ancients have told us. For example, tradition has never told us plainly whether planets are stronger in their own signs in the sense of being when thus placed more powerful both for good and evil, or whether they are stronger in the sense of being inclined to benefic action. So far as accidents are concerned, Table I seems to answer this question.

Thus statistics are a critique of tradition and sometimes, as in Table III, seem to offer very pungent criticism.

In so far as astrologers have often been too prone to interpret maps according to their own bias, making the wish the father to the thought and finding what they wanted to find, statistical investigation is a valuable corrective.

Moreover, it will stimulate inquiry, for often statistics reveal an apparent fact for which tradition seems to offer no explanation : thus, we shall be stimulated to find the reason for what seems to be a truth.

Statistics are weak in that, unless they can be spread over many lands and long periods of time, they may always be attacked on the grounds that they reflect only local or temporal conditions. Astrology stresses this weakness, because it teaches that places and times have their own specific astrological characteristics, and all births that take place within the limits of such times and places must be affected by these. For example, I may find that in my cases Mars in 0° Pisces has a certain effect. But it may be that if most of my maps are drawn from a certain country or belong to a certain epoch, this significance of Mars in 0° Pisces is really based, not on anything permanent, but upon the fact that (to take a random and hypothetical case) in the horoscope for that country or that period of time another body occupies 0° Pisces. Suppose that in the map for England, as a nation, Mars were in 0° Pisces on the cusp of the 3rd, then it would naturally follow that, in a number of maps for this country, planets in 0° Pisces might seem to indicate accidents on short journeys ; and, indeed, they would indicate this ; but it might be found that in maps for the United States there was no such significance. This, then, is a drawback to statistics, and we must suspect statistical facts unless we can see a reason for them, or unless we can spread our data over wide periods of time and over different lands.

Again, statistics are artificial. They treat of isolated horoscopic facts, whereas in actuality there is no such isolation.

I would wish the reader to bear these remarks in mind and not to suppose that, in using statistics, I am desirous of claiming more regard for them than I actually want to claim. Nor, on the other hand, do I think they are to be lightly disregarded.

The second part of the book is concerned with different classes of accident, and it is in the main carried out on conventional lines.

Twenty-one maps are reproduced, with brief notes. I have adhered here, as in compiling Table II in Part One, to the semi-arc system of house-division, because ninety-nine astrologers out of a hundred use it ; and, though there are some able and enthusiastic advocates of other methods, I have never found reason to abandon it. In regard to directional notes, I have used two or three of the best-known symbolical measures, and principally the 1° and ¼° increments. These seem to me to have demonstrated their use in this instance, as elsewhere, but naturally those who remain loyal to the older methods can easily calculate directions according to their favourite systems, and can compare the results with those that the symbolics have afforded.

With these remarks I conclude my Introduction, and trust that readers will be as kind to this as to my other astrological efforts.

CHARLES E. O. CARTER.

January, 1932.

NOTE TO SECOND EDITION

THE first edition of this work was ill-fated, for after a few hundred copies had been sold, the remainder were destroyed in the bombing of London.

Since then there has been a fairly constant demand for copies and I have decided to issue a fresh edition under the auspices of the magazine *Astrology*, to which all profits will accrue.

No important alterations have been made.

CHARLES E. O. CARTER

1961

This Second Edition of *The Astrology of Accidents* is the property of the Astrological Lodge of the Theosophical Society of Great Britain and its distribution is in the hands of the Editor of the quarterly magazine *Astrology*, to whom all inquiries and orders should be sent.

Address: 70, Gravel Hill, Addington, Croydon, Surrey.

PART ONE

ACCIDENTS IN GENERAL

§I. PRELIMINARY CONSIDERATIONS

THERE can be no question as to the importance of the subject of which this work treats. Nothing is more difficult, in the present state of our knowledge, than to diagnose in what events and circumstances any given aspect will express itself. For example, such an aspect as the Sun in opposition to Saturn may result in depressing environmental conditions due to the misfortunes or character of the father or some other person occupying an analogous position in relation to the native; or it may indicate a fall, a disease, loss of status or money, a temperamental defect (such as cowardice), an intellectual inhibition (such as fatalistic tendencies), or the loss of offspring; or perhaps it may operate in several of these ways.

But, granting this last possibility, it still remains true that some people are peculiarly liable to accidents ; their afflictions seem to tend in this direction, rather than to disease or some other expression. On the other hand, a person may have a bad Saturn, for example, which has never appeared in the form of a fall or other Saturnian form of accident, always working out in some other way, such as depression of spirits, or in a figurative fall, such as that of the ex-Kaiser William II, who had Sun opposed to Saturn, and fell from his throne.

This work represents an attempt to ascertain the astrological indications of the accident-diathesis, if we may call it so. At this point we may state definitely that the aphorisms and rules that have been handed down to us from the ancients on this question may be ruthlessly thrown aside as worthless, or nearly so.

We must first of all attempt to define an accident. I would say that it is " a bodily mishap occasioned without intent either on the part of the sufferer or the agent (if any) inflicting it."

This seems simple ; but there are numerous border-line cases. For instance, we commonly might say that a man was accidentally killed by a bull or by being thrown from a horse. But in such cases the bull certainly, and the horse probably, meant to inflict injury. Again, a street-accident may be due to such gross rashness on the part of a pedestrian or a motorist as almost to make the injury intentional. Or, if a man is blown up in war on a battleship, we should not call it an accident, but if he were fatally injured playing foot-ball we should call it one : yet in both cases the victim volunteers to meet certain risks, and, whether he does it for sport or for glory, the choice is still deliberate : hence I reject all cases of death on active service or of death or injury when a clear risk is willingly incurred. Another case of this type is death while flying, at least in the early days when this pursuit was recognisedly perilous.

We admit the fact of these gradations of accident when we talk of a " pure accident " in contrast to an accident due to carelessness. A pure accident might be exemplified by injuries from falling tiles, chimney-pots, or branches ; but even in these cases there might be some imprudence, supposing a person ventured forth in a great storm.

From these considerations the reader will see that

the subject is not a very easy one, or one that admits of strict demarcation.

Many other possible classifications may be used besides one based on the psychological conditions of the victim and the agent.

Thus we might have classifications based on :

1. Nature of instrument inflicting hurt, as knife, fire, hot water, tram or other road-vehicle, gas, and so forth.

2. Whether the hurt is self-inflicted or due to another —e.g. one might cut one's self or might be cut by another.

3. Part of body hurt.

4. Psychological reaction—e.g. whether resentful, painful, numbing, *et cetera*.

5. Extent of injury, whether fatal, slight, lasting, or temporary.

Our first investigations must be directed to discover, if possible, any factors that are *common to all serious accidents*, or at least occur more frequently than mere probability would explain.

My total collection, at the time of " closing the lists" for the tables, comprised 168 cases. These may be roughly divided as follows : asphyxiation 5, drowning 14, burns 19, scalds 9, gunshots 4, blows 21, crushings 9, wounds and cuts 7, vehicular 22, falls 32, machinery 5, railway 3, poisons 1, explosions 4, miscellaneous 10, animals 3. Some of this book was written before all of these had come to hand, hence the above figures may not exactly agree with others given in Part Two, which also contains cases that came in after the tables had been finished. Tables I and II are based on the total of 168, but Table III on only 120.

Over 100 of these cases are British, and of the rest most are from the United States. Nearly all are of modern birth.

Some, of course, have suffered from several forms of accident ; but in such cases I have taken the more serious mishaps, and have referred across to them from other sections where there seemed a good reason for so doing.

With regard to the sufficiency or otherwise of these numbers, it appears to me undeniable that useful results may be deduced from them, although, in order to obtain an exact ratio, it would be necessary to employ perhaps ten times as many, and even then the result would be subject to the limitations mentioned on page 10. But when we see such divergencies as Sun in Taurus-Sagittarius, 41 times, and Sun in Capricorn-Aquarius, 16 times, we can surely say that this suggests a strong probability that the former positions occur with greater frequency than the latter ! If, further, we say that this assumption is supported by tradition, inasmuch as the Saturn signs are said to be prudent, and Sagittarius and Taurus are respectively regarded as adventurous and careless and obstinate and self-willed, we then have a twofold foundation for our thesis. It is clear that when statistics produce a result that appears to have no traditional support, we ought to demand a very strong statistical case ; but if statistics and tradition concur, then we need not exact so high a statistical frequency. Tradition, as a rule, is founded on principles, for it was in this way that astrological knowledge has been handed down ; not till modern times has the statistical method been developed ; our fore-runners neither could nor desired to use such a process.

In studying sign-positions, we cannot usefully tabulate the slower bodies, but have included Saturn. Thus, with the ascendant, we have 8 factors, which, in 168 cases, yield 1,344 data. In studying mundane positions we have used 9 bodies, the ascendant being naturally omitted, whilst it has not seemed desirable to use Pluto, which was discovered after much of the compilation of this book had been completed. Pluto introduces a particularly difficult problem by reason of its excessive latitude. This may cause the body of the planet to be in a different house from the zodiacal degree which it occupies.

In the great majority of cases used in these tables, Pluto is not far from Neptune.

In regard to the ascending signs in Table I, it is essential to bear in mind the fact of oblique ascension, which causes Aries, for example, to rise at London in about 52 minutes, whilst Libra takes almost three hours. It is not easy to see how this can be dealt with, for, although we can apply a levelling factor if all births are at approximately the same latitude, we cannot even then be sure that our result is of value, for this would presuppose that births, on an average, occur at equal intervals throughout the day. But this has never, to my knowledge, been proved. I have therefore refrained from an attempt to adjust the ascendant-data, and must ask the student merely to bear the above fact in mind when considering them. Thus it is not as striking as it would seem at first sight that four signs (♒ ♓ ♈ ♉) have only 32 cases out of 168, the average being 56. For, in the countries from which most of my data came, these signs rise rapidly. Still, Aries = 5 does contrast in an interesting manner with Leo-Sagittarius = 48.

TABLE I

Showing the Sign-Positions of the Ascendant, Lights, and Five Planets in 168 Cases of Accidents of all Kinds.

	♈	♉	♊	♋	♌	♍	♎	♏	♐	♑	♒	♓
Asc.	5	8	9	16	24	15	22	17	25	8	8	11
☉	17	22	13	10	15	17	10	17	19	9	7	12
☽	15	10	16	17	12	13	12	14	15	14	14	16
☿	21	16	12	11	10	14	15	18	16	15	7	13
♀	17	17	8	14	12	11	14	13	22	12	11	17
♂	13	14	11	17	14	20	12	18	17	14	7	11
♃	12	10	11	16	13	11	16	14	15	13	16	21
♄	12	11	9	13	15	10	17	15	14	20	14	18
TOTALS Above Average	112			114	116		118	126	142			119
Below Average		108	89			111				105	84	

The total number of points is 1,344 and the average for each sign is 112. The highest is seen to be Sagittarius and the lowest is Aquarius. About 8 totals are so close to the mean as to have no significance.

The average for each planet is 14 a sign, the highest incidence (omitting ascendant) being 22 (☉ ♉, ♀ ♐) and the lowest 7, which occurs several times.

The highest incidence for each factor is printed in heavy type.

For the two latter take together about six times as long to rise as the first, but they occur almost ten times as often. And this although Aries would, *primâ facie*, be dubbed a sign liable to accidents !

It must be borne in mind that a very distinctive characterisation can scarcely be expected for accident-maps as such, for it is difficult to find any common factor either factual or psychological, for *all* accidents, except the negative one of absence of intention. When specific types of accident are considered, one may legitimately expect clear characteristics.

Further, we may not be surprised if sign-positions are relatively of little value in this matter, for they are generally understood to influence character more than circumstance, and, even with the Moon, they are common to too many births at the same period to be sharply distinctive of such things as grave accidents, which are exceptional. Yet we shall see that the sign-position of even the slow-moving Saturn seems to have significance in this regard—more so, indeed, than that of some faster-moving bodies, e.g. the Moon, which hardly departs from the mean.

§ 2. SIGN-POSITION

On the preceding page is printed Table I, which shows the sign-position incidence of our 168 cases.

The ascendant must be considered without forgetting the fact of long and short ascension. The infrequency of Aries and the frequency of Libra are perhaps the most noteworthy and unexpected features of the ascending signs. Aries and Pisces rise in about the same time at London, but the Martian sign has less than half as many occurrences as the Jovian. Libra outnumbers Virgo and Scorpio, though these are associated with the 6th and 8th houses, of which the second, at any rate, is somewhat suggestive of accidents. That Leo should be high is, to me at least, surprising. It is also a common ascendant in infantile mortality cases. Capricorn is a rare ascendant, and when it meets with accidents they are very seldom its own fault. This agrees with tradition, which describes the sign as sure-footed and alert.

The Sun's position (and that also of the inferior planets) must be considered in the light of the fact of more frequent births in spring-time. Nevertheless the great contrast between Sun-Taurus = 22 and Sun-Cancer = 10 might give the orthodox scientific sceptic something to account for. The high incidences in Aries, Virgo, Scorpio, and Sagittary are all rather as might be expected, except perhaps Virgo. As with the ascendant, the Saturn signs are low.

The Moon is so level as to suggest no comment except that of the negative value of the lunar influence in regard to the subject of our investigation. It is, however, rather strange that its maximum should fall in its own sign.

Mercury shows a not unexpected maximum in the two Mars signs; it has often been remarked that he is more afflicted by Mars than by Saturn. He, like Sun and ascendant, is at his minimum in Aquarius.

Venus registers one of the highest maxima in the whole table in Sagittarius, and has a minimum in Gemini that is less than a third of her maximum.

Otherwise she is near the mean. She does not follow the solar incidence, as she might have been expected to do, since they often occupy the same sign.

Mars rises high in his own sign Scorpio, but has his maximum in Virgo, owing, I think, to the special frequency with which Mars-Virgo occurs in certain classes of mishap, presently to be examined. He, again, is low in Aquarius, but otherwise shows no striking departures.

Jupiter has a maximum in his own sign Pisces, but else is close to the average.

Saturn is also high in his own sign and has a second-maximum in Pisces; otherwise he is not far from average.

Some interesting observations might be founded on this table. Taking the lights and five planets, it is noteworthy that they have maxima in different signs, Gemini, Leo, Libra, Scorpio, and Aquarius having no maxima. The Moon, Jupiter, and Saturn have maxima in their own (traditional) signs and Mars has a close second-maximum in Scorpio. One is tempted to ask why three bodies, the Sun, Mercury, and Venus, entirely break away from this rule: does the Sun really rule Taurus, Mercury rule Aries, and Venus rule Sagittarius? Each of these signs shows a 50 per cent. maximum, which is fairly substantial.

That planets are not strong in their own signs in a favourable sense is clearly demonstrated from this table. There is not a single planet which is particularly low in its own sign, and, as we have seen, three bodies have maxima in the signs they rule, and Mars is near thereto.

Nor is there any reason to think that exaltations have

any benefic effect so far as accidents go. Moon-Taurus is low ; the others call for no comment.

The establishment (so far as this table carries weight) of this important fact appears to me to justify, by itself, all the work that the compiling of the figures has demanded.

Comments on the totals appear below the table. It is not very strange that Scorpio-Sagittarius is high, or that the agile Gemini is low, but I do not know why Aquarius is so loved by the gods so far as accidents are concerned.

The totals may be analysed in several ways.

The four quadrants yield :

♈ ♉ ♊ .	. 309
♋ ♌ ♍ .	. 341
♎ ♏ ♐ .	.. 386
♑ ♒ ♓ .	. 308

As the average is 336, there are some deviations that are perhaps of interest. One might expect the third triad to be high, since it includes the signs related to the 7th house (open enemies), the 8th (death), and the 9th (adventures abroad).

The elements are :

Fire .	. 370
Air .	. 291
Earth .	. 324
Water .	. 359

The average is still 336 and the results are not surprising, since one would suppose fire to be high and air low ; and that the two others are near the mean, but

that water is somewhat in excess of earth, is what might
be expected for psychological reasons.

The qualities are :

Cardinal	. 449
Fixed .	. 434
Common	. 461

The divergence here is remarkable only for its exiguity. This surprised me ; I expected to see the common quadruplicity high, as the common signs are often flustered and maladroit when in difficult conditions and menaced with an accident. But the cardinals are near the mean throughout, only Capricorn being rather low. The fixed are high in Scorpio but very low in Aquarius. The common are high in the Jovian signs but low in the Mercurial. Thus there is, on the whole, a negative result in terms of the quadruplicities.

Taking the rulerships, we have :

Cancer-Leo .	. 230
Gemini-Virgo	. 200
Taurus-Libra	. 226
Aries-Scorpio	. 238
Sag.-Pisces .	. 261
Cap.-Aquarius	. 189

The average = 228, so that Saturn and Mercury signs are low, Jovian signs are high, and Sun-Moon and Mars signs are average. I should have expected the Mercurial signs to have been high, for I imagined them to be careless and awkward under affliction. Jupiter, though named the preserver, is unfortunately often destructive, because of his love of hazards.

How far can these figures be used in practice ? Can we build a bridge between statistics and the actual delineation of a map ?

I have before me the data of a sailor drowned in the U.S.S. S 51 disaster. Data are given on page 53, but the case came too late to be used in the table. What will be the result of applying the table to it ? I have typed this query before examining the map ; proceeding to study it, I find that there is no position below the average of 14, and all but two are above the average, the total being 129 against 114 average. This total is arrived at by taking from Table I the figures under each position that occurs in the sailor's map. Thus, as he has ☉ ♏, we take 17, ♃ ♎ 16, and so make up a " score." It will thus be clear that this case does show, in the light of the statistics of the table, a liability to accidents, or at least it does not contradict the possibility of such an eventuality.

On the whole, tables such as this are probably of most practical use on the negative side : by comparing a given map with the table, it may be possible to say that an accident is highly unlikely, but even a high average would not *alone* imply an accident, which, in the end, must depend upon aspects.

We have said that a weak point in statistical work is that it artificially dissects a map which actually exists as a whole and has no real meaning except as a whole. Thus we may say that certain positions, as given above, incline to accidents. But such positions are shown in an isolation, in which they never exist. Sun in Taurus may be prone to accidents, but we cannot really study such a configuration, except artificially : in practical astrology it will always occur in combination with a house-position, and probably with various aspects. Again, the table shows that Sun-Taurus is bad and Venus-Sagittarius is bad, but it does not show whether or not these two positions *together* are bad : they might conceivably operate to cancel each other, as two noxious germs in the human body might do.

In paying all due attention to statistics we must nevertheless not be blind to the limitations of such methods.

§ 3. HOUSE-POSITION

TABLE II gives the results of an examination of 168 cases.

Though the compilation took considerable time, the lessons that may be learnt can be perceived at a glance.

Firstly, the houses as such are mostly near the average total of 126. The exceptions are the 4th and 12th, which are high, although the former does not hold the maximum of any body ; and the 2nd, which is low. The other nine are too near to the average to be of any interest.

The Moon and Venus are very level frequencies, but the Moon rises to 21 in the 7th, and Venus, curiously, has her maximum in the 1st.

Sun, Mercury, and Mars have maxima of 21, but have no striking minima. All three have secondary maxima in the 12th.

Jupiter does not rise very high or fall very low, the lowest (9) and the highest (19) being no very wide deviations from the mean.

On the other hand, Saturn, Uranus, and Neptune

TABLE II

Showing the House-Positions of the Lights and Seven Planets according to the Semi-Arc System, with 5° Orbs, in 168 Cases of Accidents.

	I	II	III	IV	V	VI	VII	VIII	IX	X	XI	XII
☉	12	10	**21**	17	15	11	11	11	14	12	15	19
☽	12	12	12	16	16	14	**21**	14	10	15	14	12
☿	10	14	**21**	17	10	8	14	15	12	14	13	20
♀	**17**	14	14	16	16	13	8	15	13	12	15	15
♂	**21**	14	11	17	15	14	10	11	9	13	14	19
♃	15	9	15	15	15	11	13	**19**	13	17	13	13
♄	8	10	12	18	12	20	9	14	15	11	**23**	16
♅	**22**	15	16	16	14	16	7	8	13	17	12	12
♆	8	3	9	12	16	5	**23**	17	21	15	16	**23**
TOTALS Over Average			131	144	129					126	135	149
Below Average	125	101				112	116	124	120			

Total data, 1,512 ; average per house for each body, 14 ; average total for each house, 126.

(as if to compensate for the fact that by reason of slow motion their sign-positions lose distinctiveness) show extremely interesting results. Both Saturn and Neptune have very low frequencies in the first quadrant (♄ – 30, ♆ – 20). Saturn rises to 23 in the 11th, and Neptune to a like figure in both 7th and 12th, so that these two houses have more than a third the total for this planet. Uranus, on the other hand, has his highest frequency in the 1st, like Mars, whilst his lowest is in the 7th, so that he is almost the reverse of Neptune, whose lowest, 3, is in the 2nd but who is also low in the 1st.

This minimum of 3 is the lowest in the table, whilst Neptune is also low in the 6th—5 occurrences. There is no other minimum below 7.

It therefore seems as if Neptune is particularly important in accidents ; this would seem to be the legitimate deduction from the abrupt variations in its house-incidence.

If we wish to test this table by reference to the case that was used on page 26 with the sign-positions, we can tabulate the " score " as follows :

☉ in	3rd	=	21
☽	10th	=	15
☿	3rd	=	21
♀	2nd	=	14
♂	3rd	=	11
♃	2nd	=	9
♄	3rd	=	12
♅	3rd	=	16
♆	10th	=	15
	Total	=	134 against the average
			of 126

The Sun and Mercury are in their maxima and only 3 are below the mean.

§ 4. ASPECTS.

IN order to examine these I have tabulated the distances (or elongations) between certain bodies which might be presumed to play an important part in accidents, using 120 cases.

In this connection it is, however, necessary to point out that, for astronomical reasons, certain distances occur more often than others, quite apart from the nature of the horoscopes under review.

I am indebted to Mr. K. E. Krafft, for the following data relating to this fact :

" The conjunction between the Sun and Mars is found about three times more frequently than the opposition. For more accurate data see *Sterne und Mensch*, 1928–1929, various papers by Dr. Kritzinger. For the Sun and Jupiter the angles around the conjunction are found about 15 per cent. more frequently than the mean number would be. For Saturn it is about 8 per cent., for Uranus about 5 per cent., and for Neptune about 3 per cent. The displacement of the Moon being comparatively great, no practically important deviation from the norm takes place. As regards Mercury and Mars in relation to Saturn, no general formula can be given, because of strange periodicities in their movements. In such cases the best way is to calculate, from the ephemeris of the years concerned, a normal frequency distribution by taking, e.g. the angles for every 10th day. You will then see how irregular a ' pure chance distribution ' can become, and this may give you a hint to be cautious when interpreting the results of your statistics."

I gladly pass on Mr. Krafft's admonition to my readers, whilst observing that, subject to its being remembered, even a number such as is here employed may not be valueless, although it cannot be regarded as sufficing to prove exact ratios.

In the following Table III the elongations are tabulated in 5° areas, from 0° to 180°. Figures of 7 or over are in heavy type, and totals of 6 are also so printed when they fall in an area adjacent to another 6 or any higher number, so that they may be deemed to form one extended area together.

The average of each 5° area is of course $3\frac{1}{3}$.

Area ending:	5°	10°	15°	20°	25°	30°	35°	40°	45°	50°	55°	60°	65°	70°	75°	80°	85°	90°
☉ – ♂	8	4	9	13	3	5	5	4	3	5	4	2	1	5	2	5	2	1
☉ – ♄	1	1	3	4	2	3	3	2	3	5	5	2	2	10	5	3	3	3
☉ – ♅	2	2	1	4	3	6	3	2	6	5	5	2	3	5	4	3	4	1
☉ – ♆	2	8	7	4	4	5	3	2	4	1	5	6	7	2	3	1	3	1
☽ – ♂	4	5	2	8	4	8	4	5	4	4	0	4	3	3	4	5	3	3
☽ – ♄	7	0	4	4	3	1	0	3	5	4	5	5	2	3	3	3	2	8
☽ – ♅	2	1	5	7	2	3	4	8	2	3	3	3	4	2	3	6	2	4
☽ – ♆	2	2	2	4	3	5	0	3	2	5	2	4	4	6	6	2	2	1
☿ – ♂	9	10	7	6	5	6	5	3	3	6	3	4	1	2	3	5	0	2
☿ – ♄	4	2	2	5	2	4	4	3	2	4	0	3	5	0	2	5	6	7
☿ – ♅	2	1	6	5	3	0	7	3	4	2	3	5	3	4	3	3	2	4
☿ – ♆	5	5	6	5	4	2	3	2	4	4	3	4	2	5	4	2	4	2
♂ – ♄	5	1	2	2	2	4	5	2	1	2	2	7	6	3	4	6	4	4
♂ – ♅	9	1	2	0	3	4	4	5	7	2	5	2	3	4	6	4	1	3
♂ – ♆	4	0	2	3	0	8	1	5	4	3	6	6	3	7	3	3	2	2
♄ – ♅	1	5	5	4	5	7	1	4	2	6	5	3	2	1	3	4	0	3
♄ – ♆	1	4	0	7	1	6	5	3	0	4	5	4	4	3	2	0	3	3
	68	52	65	85	49	77	57	59	56	65	61	66	55	65	60	60	43	52

TOTAL: 2,040 : Average per 5° Area : 56⅔.

III
Elongations of the Bodies Stated.

95°	100°	105°	110°	115°	120°	125°	130°	135°	140°	145°	150°	155°	160°	165°	170°	175°	180°
4	3	0	0	0	4	3	6	4	4	0	0	2	2	0	1	2	4
1	5	**9**	**6**	4	4	3	2	2	3	4	1	4	2	3	2	2	3
5	3	1	3	4	**8**	1	**7**	5	4	3	2	3	2	1	1	5	1
5	2	2	3	6	3	1	2	3	5	3	1	2	1	4	3	4	2
1	1	4	1	2	2	4	3	2	3	2	4	4	3	3	2	3	3
4	3	2	5	1	6	2	1	3	2	3	4	4	**7**	4	1	2	4
1	2	4	4	4	3	3	4	5	3	3	5	0	1	3	**7**	3	1
5	2	4	3	5	1	3	**6**	**7**	**8**	2	1	1	2	4	**7**	3	1
1	3	3	3	2	3	3	1	0	2	3	1	3	3	3	1	2	3
3	**8**	2	4	3	**6**	**7**	1	2	3	4	1	1	3	3	4	3	2
7	**7**	3	2	0	5	1	4	**6**	**7**	3	3	2	3	1	2	3	1
4	2	3	3	2	**7**	3	3	2	2	5	2	0	1	**7**	3	2	3
5	4	4	4	6	2	1	1	3	3	**7**	2	3	2	2	5	3	1
3	2	2	4	**10**	3	0	5	2	5	2	1	3	5	3	2	3	0
2	1	5	2	4	5	4	4	5	2	3	1	3	3	2	3	5	4
3	1	6	1	5	0	1	2	6	3	6	2	**7**	3	6	3	1	3
6	1	2	3	4	1	6	2	5	5	4	5	3	1	3	2	**6**	**6**
60	50	56	51	62	63	46	54	62	64	57	36	45	44	52	49	52	42

TOTALS IN TABLE III GRAPHICALLY REPRESENTED

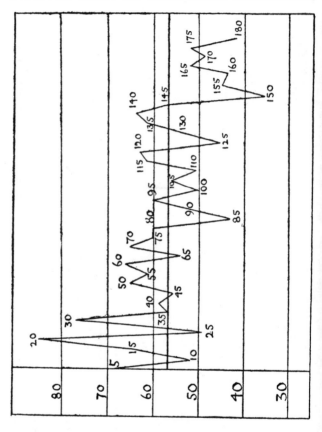

List of Principal Stresses extracted from Table III.

Sun-Mars	0–5, 10–20.
Saturn	65–70, 100–110.
Uranus	115–120, 125–130.
Neptune	5–15, 55–65.

Moon-Mars	15–20, 25–30.
Saturn	0–5, 85–90, 155–160.
Uranus	15–20, 35–40, 165–170.
Neptune	65–75, 125–140, 165–170.

Mercury-Mars	0–20.
Saturn	80–90, 95–100, 115–125.
Uranus	30–35, 90–100, 130–140.
Neptune	115–120, 160–165.

Mars-Saturn	55–65, 140–145.
Uranus	0–5, 40–45, 110–115.
Neptune	25–30, 50–60, 65–70.

| Saturn-Uranus | 25–30, 150–155. |
| Neptune | 15–20, 170–180. |

Two outstanding features occur in this table.

Firstly, it is observable that the emphasised areas, or *stresses*, fall differently—almost entirely differently— with each pair of planets.

Secondly, the stresses fall very differently from the recognised aspects. For instance, the area 85°–95°, covering the square, is noticeably weak, despite the traditional belief that nothing is more conducive to accidents than the squares of certain bodies. Again, in general the opposition is very weak, and even the conjunction is not consistently high.

It is not my present purpose to discuss the theoretical purport of these facts, and it may be suggested that a much larger tabulation should precede any such investigation. But one question of immense possible importance thrusts itself upon us : supposing that these results are correct, even in an approximate sense, and that they represent the aspectual conditions causing accidents ; are they also valid in relation to other occurrences and conditions, or *must we suppose that, as each pair of bodies has its own stresses, so again each class of human contingency has its appropriate stresses true in regard to itself but inapplicable to other classes ?*

This would mean, in plain English, that there would be separate sets of stresses for each pair of bodies and for each class of conditions.

Such a possibility opens vistas of complexity that only prolonged and patient research could unravel. As regards the traditional aspects, I think we shall require much evidence before we desert them, and certainly few will impugn their validity so far as psychological astrology is concerned, even if in some respects we have to alter our valuations. Disease, I am inclined to think, has its own " stresses," different both from Table III and from the conventional aspects. In 25 cases of cancer there is the very high number of 6 incidences between 70° and 80° for the Sun-Jupiter elongation. In the same 25 cases there are also 6 Jupiter-Saturn elongations between 52° and 58°—a very narrow area indeed. In 32 cases of consumption there are 7 cases wherein the Sun-Neptune elongation is between 100° and 106°, again a narrow area.

One may be permitted some satisfaction in noting that there are far fewer stresses in Table III than there are traditional bad aspects. These last, using conventional orbs, cover about a third of the ecliptic ; that is to say, if a planet is in any one point of the zodiac it will throw adverse rays to about a third of the circle. But in Table III each pair has usually two stresses covering each about 5° to 10°, so that, using the whole 360° of the circle instead of 180°, as in the table, we have at most 40° under adverse influence, instead of about 120°. Thus life, in regard to accidents, is not as black as it is painted by traditional astrology !

Reverting to the table and graph, we shall perhaps be most struck by the general tendency of the totals to exceed the mean or to fall but little below it up to 80°, after which there is a distinct tendency to drop. From 145° to the end the line is entirely beneath the average-line, though the quincunx and opposition fall in these areas. From 175° to 180° is the lowest area except only 145°-150°. Some of the changes are very abrupt, as from the maximum of 85 between 15° and 20° and the fall to 49 in the next area. Contrasting a minimum of 36 with an apex of 85, based on so many cases, we cannot consider any suggestion that these results are fortuitous and without significance, although it must be acknowledged that, on a much larger total, they might, and no doubt would, be modified in detail.

It may be noticed, however, that though these totals and the graph based thereon are of striking interest, they are misleading from a practical point of view, because even the most marked divergences are not true of all planetary pairs. Thus the apex 15°-20° does not occur at all between Mars and Uranus. The only columns that contain no stresses are 20°-25°, 45°-50°, 50°-55°, 75°-80°, and 145°-150°; and it may be surmised that these also would disappear in a table of all possible planetary contacts.

As to the rationale of the incidence of these maxima and minima I hazard no conjecture at all, though several possible astronomical explanations may occur to those more mathematically minded that I am. Suggestions have been made that a class of aspects may be related to the apparent speeds of the planets,[1] but this does not seem to be the case here. For example, Neptune is stationary at an elongation of 100° from the Sun, but there is no corresponding stress in Table III. On the other hand, I do not think that the points of maximum velocity are stressed either.

[1] See letter by Mr. Stanley Gritton, *Astrology*, autumn number, 1930, referring to *The Horoscope* for October 1903.

Part Two

EXAMPLES OF PARTICULAR FORMS OF ACCIDENTS

NOTE

Such cases as are printed with the erected horoscope of births are called *Examples*, and are referred to throughout by that name for distinction's sake. All other data are referred to as *Cases*, and either have their references according to their sources, if they have already been published, or else, if they have not before appeared in print, are given serial reference-numbers according to the type of accident to which they belong, thus, D = drowning, SC = scalding, BL = blows.

The examples and cases do not comprise all the maps that I have used : for various reasons I have not thought fit to publish more than a selection.

Readers are warmly invited to send reliable data of accidents, especially of such kinds as are not well represented in this collection, as, for example, injuries from animals. These will be filed for the purpose of being incorporated in future editions.

INTRODUCTORY NOTE

IN this portion of the book I desire to give data and examples of fifteen classes of accident, with a short discussion of the probable general characteristics of each class, together with a concise examination of the examples given.

It might appear logical to continue in this part what has been begun in Part One, and to base all discussion and investigation on the results that are summed up in the three tables. But this would be a complete break with traditional astrology, and would constitute a much bolder step than the results already given would justify. Therefore it will be found that Part Two is substantially based on traditional astrology, although I have appended to the examples brief references to the tables, for interest's sake.

It will be found that I have printed 21 erected horoscopes ; and in all there are data for some 160 cases, most of which have never before, to my knowledge, been published. Thus those who wish to continue the study of the astrology of accidents will have a considerable store of material upon which to draw.

Brief notes have been added to the examples on the directional influences at the time of accident. In this connection I have used only symbolic measures, believing them to be superior to the primary and secondary systems of the past, though, of course, students who differ from me on this head can easily work the directions for the cases upon which they are engaged according to whatever system they favour.

The measures employed are the 4/7ths, the one-degree, and the slower but very useful $\frac{1}{4}°$ and $\frac{1}{8}°$. In the main I have used the one-degree.

§ 5. ASPHYXIATION

CASES for study are :

N.N. 77, 270, S.D. p. 71, 2 Exx. hereunder.

The following cases of suicide by asphyxiation are of interest for comparison, since there are not available many cases of accidents of this class :

SU 1—Male, 6.30 p.m., 4.6.1906, Damascus, Syria, death 28.1.31.

SU 2—Male, 7.30 p.m., 1.1.1914, New England, death 19.1.1930.

SU 3—Male, 6.30 p.m., 27.10.1895, Geneva, death 15.9.1905.

In these suicidal cases note the afflictions in the vicinity of 13° of the common signs, also from Saturn.

I do not know if the two N.N. cases given above are known to have been accidental or were of a doubtful character. Zola's case does not suggest suicide, as Saturn is rather well placed.

S.D. p. 71, is an instance of carelessness ; and characteristically the chief affliction is undoubtedly ☉ ☍ ♂ , the fact that it is separating being probably responsible for the life of the native having been preserved. Here there can be no question that the particular manner in which this contact worked out was due to the heavy ♊ ♐ oppositions, including Pluto in 14° ♊ , ♀ being ruler of the 8th.

Observe that PL–♄ afflictions occur also in the two cases below. But in this case the ♊ ♐ oppositions do not fall so far forward in the two signs as in the cases that follow.

Example No. 1

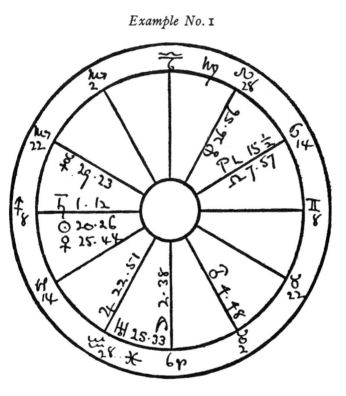

Female born 7 a.m., December 13, 1926, 51°N., 2°W. Died August 12, 1930. After being put to bed she played with matches ; the bedclothes caught fire, and she was suffocated. When found, the lower part of the body had been badly burnt by the smouldering sheets.

Psychological Considerations

We can, under this head, examine the map for (*a*) mischievousness and (*b*) love of playing with fire—though this is a common childish habit.

♐ rising and ♂ in 5th seem sufficient to account for both features, but we may also add ☽ and ☿ in ♂ signs. ♃, the ruler, is in close par. with ♂. Though ♄, the planet of caution, is not very severely afflicted, its prudential action would scarcely operate strongly at such an early age.

Circumstantial Considerations

Why fire and why suffocation ?

The first question seems answered by the presence of 6 out of 11 points (lights, 8 planets, and ascendant) being in the fiery trigon.

As regards asphyxiation, we cannot ask for clearer indications than the opposition of ♃ to ♅, both □ ☿ and both part-rulers of the 3rd, whilst Uranus, in that house, receives two potent squares from the 1st—note that the accident was entirely self-occasioned. ♊ was certainly untenanted, but note ☿ ☌ ♄, a common indication of suffocative conditions. If it be said that the Moon, ruling the 8th, is unafflicted, I would point to a parallel to Uranus, and also to its being in square to the Nodes—a most unfortunate position.

The Kennison reaction points show some severe afflictions. [1]

---

[1] The theory of these reaction points postulates for every body in the horoscope a point that is as far from its planet as 0° ♈ is from the ascendant. In this case, for example, 0° ♈ is 112° from the ascendant ; hence each planet has a point that is 112° from itself, in the sense of the zodiac. Thus the reaction point of ♂ (abbreviated rpt. ♂) is ☌ ♅ and rpt. ♅ is ☌ ☉.

Tables

There is a stress between ♂ ♅.

☿ occupies a bad house, and the ascendant ♐ is also, as we have seen, exceptionally prone to accidents.

Directions

In so young a child it might be argued that these can hardly be traced, yet there is a series of o-d directions, viz. ♄ ⚹ ♂, ♃ ∠ ♆, ♆ □ ♄, ☽ □ Nodes ; ♅ is certainly △ ☿, which is too weak to save.

Point of life is square to Pluto in the 8th. Even the slow ¼° measure yields PL ⊡ ♄ and ☿ ♂ ♄.

Example No. 2

Lady born 0.8 p.m., August 24, 1867, Washington, D.C. She became unconscious from geyser fumes in connection with a bath, at Zürich, at 9 p.m., October 30, 1927, and she was also nearly drowned in August 1899.

Circumstantial Considerations

There is once again a ☿ ♄ affliction, and Pluto is also involved, probably as a very important agent in the matter. ☿ rules the 8th and has some helpful aspects which doubtless were instrumental in preventing a fatal ending. ☽ in ♊ in 8th is characteristic ; this body is unafflicted. Baths may come under ♍ or ♏ or both, and there are ill-aspected bodies in each. Even ♎ may have a connection, for the ancients certainly recommended bathing when the Moon is in this sign.

Tables

♃ is in an unfavourable sign.

There are four severe stresses, according to Table III, namely, ☽♅, ☽♆, ☿♅, ☿♆.

Directions

The arc for the asphyxiation = 60° 11′, and we see

Example No. 2

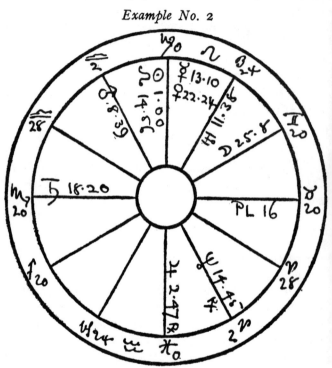

that ☿ goes to ☍ ♆, the saving element being certainly the natal trine.

As the ¼° arc = 15° 3′ there are duplicate influences, e.g. ☉ △ PL and also PL □ ☉.

The 4/7th are = 34° 22′; this yields ♂ □ ☿ and ♆ ☍ ♄—both very characteristic.

Indeed, the numerous ☿ afflictions are very noteworthy.

In order properly to describe the astrological indices of danger of death from asphyxiation it would be necessary to have far more cases than are available for my researches, yet even the above may serve as pointers in the right direction.

§ 6. DROWNING

A GOOD number of cases of drowning and of narrow escapes from the water have been published, and we may quote the following for reference :

Stanley Condor, 1.45 p.m., September 30, 1894, Cheshire.

N.N. 73, 100, 402, 198.

I remember reading that the astrologer Sepharial was almost drowned on one occasion, but I cannot trace where this note appeared.

Boy drowned on way to school, M.A. January 1917, data 7.25 a.m., April 29, 1875, Manchester.

Hartley, bandmaster of the *Titanic* and Young Lady drowned on the same ship, reference M.A. August 1912, and M.A. December 1912.[1]

D 1—" A brilliant young man " born 4 p.m., May 24, 1906, London, and drowned in a boating accident, May 1926.

D 2—Male born Croydon, near London, October 30, 1880, probable ascendant end of Pisces. Run down by

[1] Data are : Hartley : 2.6. 1878, place not stated, M.C. ♒ 28, asc. ♋ 5, ☉ ♊ 11¼, ☽ ♊ 25½, ☿ ♉ 17½, ♀ ♈ 28, ♂ ♋ 17, ♃ ♒ 7, ♄ ♈ 1½, ♅ ♌ 26, ♆ ♉ 8½, PL ♉ 25.
Young Lady : Born 7 a.m., 16.12.1891, Salisbury.

a steamer when boating and almost drowned, April 1927.

See also Exx. below, and CR 6.

In P.A., 2nd ed., p. 143, it is stated that " drowning is specially shown by afflictions involving the end of ♊ ♐ or beginnings of ♋ ♑ ; and the end of ♈ ≏ and beginnings of ♉ ♏." That is to say, afflictions to bodies near, on either side, to 0° ♋ ♑ and 0° ♉ ♏.

This thesis is well exemplified by the cases now under consideration. Mars on the line 0° ♉ ♏ seems very characteristic.

Ex. No. 3 below	♂ 1 ♏ ☍ ☽, ♆ 1 ♋ ☍ ♃.
Conder .	♂ 4 ♉, ♃ 5 ♋ □ ☉.
N.N. 100 .	♂ 1 ♉, ♅ 27 ♐.
N.N. 73 .	♄ 2 ♉, asc. 26 ♐.
N.N. 402 .	. . . , ☽ 29 ♊ ☍ ♂ 29 ♐.
N.N. 198 .	♂ 5 ♉, ☿ 5½ ♋ □ ♄.
" Boy drowned on way to school "	♆ 0° ♉, ☿ 27½ ♈ ☍ ♃, ♂ 2½ ♑.
Hartley .	♆ 8 ♉, ☽ 25½ ♊ □ ♄.
" Young Lady " (*Titanic*)	♂ ♅ 5 ♏, ☉ 24 ♐, ☽ 4 ♋.
D 1 above	. . . . , ♀ 28 ♊.
D 2 .	♂ 6 ♏, ☽ 28 ♍.

The last case but one shows afflictions in the middle of the mutables, and appears exceptional in its feature so far as drowning is concerned.

Turning to aspects, there are contacts (by no means all bad) between Mercury and Saturn in every case except the last and the " Young Lady," and even there Mercury is in Capricorn.

We have the following Neptune contacts in the eleven cases above :

1. ☍ ♃ lord 1, △ ♂ lord 4.
2. □ ♀ lady 4.
3. □ ☿ in 4, ☌ ♅ ⚻ ♄.
4. ☌ ♂ ♃, ☍ ♄ in 4.
5. ⚼ ♂ lord 4.
6. ⚹ ♂ (debilitated) lord 4.
7. ☌ ☉ lord 4.
8. ☌ ☿ ⚹ ☉, both ruling 4.
9. □ ruler.
10. □ ♄ lord 4, ☍ ♅.
11. ☍ ☉ ♂ (♂ part-lord 1st).

These seem to indicate clearly that *peril from the water is shown by an affliction of Neptune either to the ruler or to the lord or occupant of the 4th.*

However, Saturn, not Neptune, would seem to be the chief anaretic agent in drowning: we have the following chief Saturnian afflictions in the foregoing eleven cases:

1. ♄ afflicts ♀ and ♃.
2. ♄ ☌ ☽ ☿.
3. ♄ □ ☉.
4. ♄ ☍ ♂, ♃, ♆ and M.C.
5. ♄ □ ☉.
6. ♄ □ ☉ ☽ ☿.
7. ♄ ☌ ☽ (wide).
8. ♄ □ ☽.
9. ♄ □ ☉.
10. ♄ □ ☽ ♂ ♃.
11. None (native was resuscitated).

As regards the ascending signs, note that 5 out of 11 times ♐ appears on the ascendant.

It can, I think be held that the above furnish the elements of the criteria necessary to indicate danger from the water.

We will now give somewhat more detailed attention to the first of the above cases, which is Example No. 3 in the book.

Example No. 3

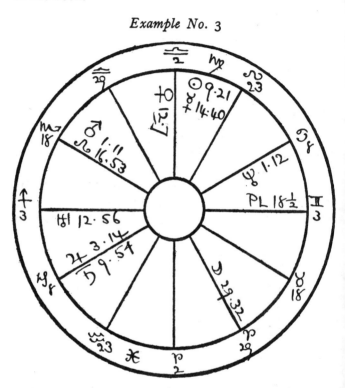

Boy born 1.30 p.m., September 2, 1901, Manchester, and drowned in the river, 12.8.1907.

Psychological Considerations

These may be taken as covered by the rising sign, by the opposition of Neptune to the ruler, and the violent ☽ ☍ ♂. There are here some elements of daring and mischief, or at any rate of error, though the last of these configurations might easily act circumstantially without any reference to the mental condition of the victim. It is notoriously difficult to tell how far any given horoscopic feature will act psychologically and how far exteriorly.

Circumstantial Considerations

We have already examined eleven cases from the standpoint of area-affliction, and afflictions from Saturn and Neptune, and we have pointed out the frequent occurrence of Sagittarius as an ascending sign. We have also mentioned the frequency of ☿ - ♄ aspects, not always evil. Here there is a trine between ☿ and ♄, but we also see ☿ □ ♅, which is rising. The ruler of the 8th is heavily afflicted by an applying aspect to the opposition of the lord of the 4th and 12th, placed in the 8th sign. Both benefics are heavily afflicted. The Sun leaves several good aspects, comes to △ ♄, and then to □ ♅ PL. ♄ is ᚆ cusp 8th.

Turning to the tables in Part One, there are, we find, three critical sign-positions, that of the ascendant, of ♂, and of ♄.

The only critical house-position is that of ♅ in 1st.

In stresses we have ☿ ♄, ♂ ♅, ♄ ♅.

Directions

Although, as in Example No. 1, the native died young, there are ample directional indications. The o-d direction ♃ △ ☉ is spoilt by the debility of ♃; there are also ♅ ᚆ PL and ♃ ♂ ♄ by the same increment.

By ¼° there are ♅ □ ☿, ♄ □ ♀, ♆ ᚆ ♃, ☽ ᚆ ♂; and by 4/7ths there is ☉ □ ♅.

♂, by transit, is in 7° ♑, afflicting all four cardinal positions.

Example No. 2 above is also a case of narrow escaping from drowning. This agrees well with the rules laid down.

We may also refer to a case of suicide by drowning, cited in V. E. Robson's *Text-Book*. Male born 7.25 p.m., December 21, 1881, Bucks. ☉ and ☽ are afflicted by ♂ at the beginning of ♑, and ☿ is □ ♄, which is in 6° ♉. We have ♃ ☌ ♅, and ♄, though in good aspect to the lights, is □ ascendant. Ruler □ ♅.

Would it be easy to say that this is a case of intentional drowning, in distinction from the other examples cited of accidental drowning? It is not a map that comes out badly from the test of Tables I and II, for ♀ ♐ is the only sign-position that is shown to be rather high, and the only house-position that is at all remarkable is ♂ 12th. There are four stresses (☽ ♅, ☿ ♅, ♂ ♄, ♂ ♅), but these stresses can hardly be restricted to accident cases only, though, as we have mentioned on page 36, it is difficult to guess how far the scope of Table III extends.

.   .   .   .

Since writing the above the following cases have come to hand :

Five children drowned in *Titanic* (brothers and sisters, hours of birth unknown) :

1. Girl, 12.3.1896
2. Boy, 22.5.1897
3. Boy, 12.8.1896
4. Girl, 16.3.1900
5. Boy, 25.9.1901

The following may have been death from drowning or from suffocation : Sailor, lost in the ramming of U.S.S. S 51 by the *City of Rome*, 10.24 p.m., September 25, 1925, born 1.15 a.m., November 10, 1897, 45° N., 93° W. Ref. Misc. 10.

§ 7. BURNS

THESE constitute a very interesting class of accident.

The following cases for study are given, in addition to three Examples below.

B 1—Female, 1.30 p.m., 28.4.1902, Geneva, extensive burns.

B 3—Female, 9.0 a.m., 1.5.1907, London, night-dress caught fire. Died 4.1.1918.

B 4—Male, 1 p.m., 19.6.1891, Birmingham, foot twice burnt while working as a moulder in an iron foundry.

B 5—Male, born about noon, 19.5.1881, Swindon, Wilts, burnt all the skin off right hand end November 1918—daughter was frying, pan caught fire, and native was burnt in snatching it from her.

B 6—Female, 1 a.m., 12.2.1893, Midlands, burnt very badly on face and neck, November or December 1899. Pinafore caught fire.

B 7—Female, 10.30 a.m. approximate, 25.8.1901, Yorkshire ; candle ignited papers in a dark cupboard which she was examining ; back, neck, and one breast burnt, in hospital for a year. Happened 18.4.1918.

B 8—Female, 10 p.m., 16.7.1877, London ; set herself on fire when nursing and both arms badly burnt.

N.N. Nos. 192, 414, 687, 812, 889.

In the investigation of burns I have used in all 19 cases, from which the above are selected.

In these cases some points stand out clearly, though I would not say that the specific indications of this class of accident are extremely plain.

Out of 19 cases the Moon occupies one or other of the last four signs in no less than 14. It occurs only twice in the first half of the zodiac, once in Aries and once in Leo (both fire). It is once in Libra and once in Scorpio.

Another feature is the frequency—not unexpected—of Martian conjunctions. Of these there are no less than 15, made up as follows: With Sun 4, Uranus 3, Saturn, Jupiter and M.C. 2 each, Neptune-Pluto and ascendant 1 each. Mercury is also involved in 2 of these 15.

The sign-position of Mars is not very irregular. It occurs in all signs except Sagittarius, and the only indications of possible maxima are Aries, Taurus, and Gemini—the first three.

The Sun-Mars elongations are very striking. Instead of the average of 90° (see, however, note on page 30) we find an average of $42\frac{1}{2}°$. In 10 cases the two bodies are within 20° and in only 3 are they over 70° apart, these three being all within orbs of the trine, with a maximum of 128°. It appears, therefore, that the conventional remote afflictions (♎, ♐, ♑) are innocuous so far as burns are concerned.

As regards conventional aspects, it might be possible to say with some truth that afflictions in common signs, with the involvement of the fire-element (either by sign or planet), are common. Moon-Saturn and Mars-Saturn afflictions are common. Neptune is a not-infrequent afflictor.

As for special areas, the following occur often, but not invariably : about 10° cardinals, 21° fire-air, and 29° fire-air. In these matters I take the orbs very narrowly—about 2°.

Example No. 4

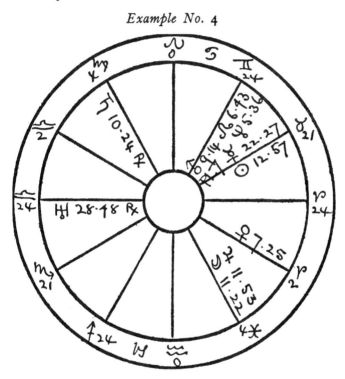

Female, born 6 p.m., May 3, 1891, Geneva ; died of burns, 2.10 a.m., May 9, 1918.

Psychological Considerations

The heavy mutable afflictions may readily be taken as indications of carelessness or maladroitness. Uranus rising is notably impatient, and the 5th house afflictions might make for imprudence, since they incline, traditionally, towards gambling and the taking of hazards in small things and great.

Circumstantial Indications

The remarks made above are fully exemplified by this map, but only the third of the three areas there mentioned is occupied, viz. ♅ 29 ♎.

Tables

Sign-positions of the Sun and Jupiter are unfavourable.

House-positions of Saturn and Uranus, likewise.

A stress occurs as follows : ☿ ♂.

Directions

The arc for death = 27° 01'.

One-degree directions are ♄ ☍ ♀ ruler 8, asc. ☍ ☿ in 8, ☽ ♃ ✳ ♂ from radical □, ⊙ ☌ ♂.

By ¼° increment we have ☿ ⊼ ♅, ♆ □ ☽ ♃.

Example No. 5

Male, born 10.50 p.m., April 8, 1902, Geneva ; died, 0.50 p.m., September 3, 1904. " Brûlures étendues."

Psychological Considerations

These can scarcely be said to arise in a child of less than 2½ years, unless through some operation of the unconscious. There are mutable afflictions, but they are less severe than in the preceding case.

Circumstantial Considerations

Again we have afflictions in common signs with some fire-element (♅ ♐), and there are ☽ ♄ if not ♂ ♄ contacts. ♆ also afflicts, and he, ♅, and ☽ occupy specified areas. 10° cardinals is unoccupied.

Example No. 5

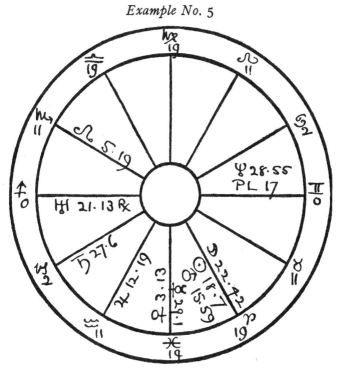

Tables

The ascendant and Saturn are unfavourable by sign, and Uranus and Neptune occupy unfavourable houses.

When we come to stresses we find a series which, if these elongations are the true, or at least the principal,

" bad aspects " in regard to accidents, would amply account for the tragic and early death of the child. There are : ☉ ♂, ☉ ♅, ☽ ♄, ☽ ♆, ☿ ♂, ☿ ♅.

Directions

It might be claimed that these would not appear in a death under an arc of 2° 25'. Nevertheless, by one degree Mars is conjunction the Sun, the ascendant is in square to Venus, and there are two quincunx aspects, which are never to be neglected or under-rated in 6th or 8th house matters, since the quincunx, taken from the ascendant, falls in or near the cusps of these houses.

By duodenary (2½°) progression Mars is close to the Moon, and by transit he was opposed to Jupiter on the day of the accident.

Example No. 6

Lady, born 8.20 a.m., September 10, 1893, Birmingham. At the age of three or four her arm and the lower part of her face were burnt, so that for a time her life was despaired of. Her pinafore caught fire from a flame caused by the draught from an open door.

Circumstantial

The conjunction Moon-Sun-Mars is a pretty clear indication of danger from fire, and although Neptune, which is in square to all three, is usually associated with water, we are inclined to give it some sort of rulership over Sagittarius, as well as over Pisces, in partnership with Jupiter, and to allow it a partly fiery action. Note also Pluto.

We have no conventional Saturn afflictions, which is unusual ; but two of the three areas are occupied.

Tables

Mars in Virgo is a weak sign-position, but the child was entirely innocent of blame.

There are some important stresses of an appropriate character : ☉ ♂ , ☿ ♂ , ♄ ♅ .

Example No. 6

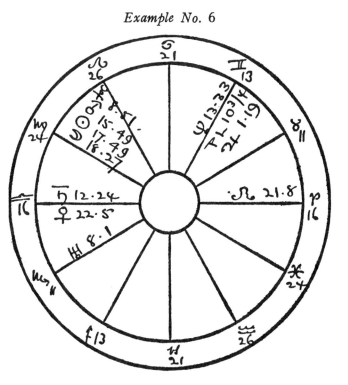

Directions

The time of the accident is not known with exactness.

. . . .

When re-typing this manuscript for press, the case of

King Victor Emmanuel II, N.N. 964, was brought to my attention in connection with burns.

It is related of this monarch that when a baby in his cradle he almost lost his life by reason of his nurse's setting fire to curtains. She saved the child, but herself died as a result of the injuries she received. Two other accidents befell, or nearly befell, him—a beam fell upon his aide-de-camp, narrowly missing him, and a warship, upon which he was taking a holiday, struck a rock and sank.

Referring to our notes on the features of the burns map, we do not find the Moon in the latter half of the zodiac, but we do see a strong Mars conjunction. Mars is in a sign which we mentioned as a possible maximum, and it is near the Sun (24°). Mars is not square the Moon, but is square the cusp 8th in Cancer, and he is trine Saturn, which good aspect may have helped to save the infant from actual harm. Jupiter occupies one of the areas. Considering there was no injury, but only danger, these indications are fairly clear. The natus, of course, is not a dangerous one.

§ 8. SCALDS

Two examples are given below, and there are the following cases for study :

SC 1—Female case from Raphael's *Private Instructions*, born 3.55 p.m., 21.8.1894, 52° 30' N. 0° W. Died 1.11.1894. Mother spilt kettle over legs and feet.

SC 2—Male, born 9 a.m., 5.10.1909, Sydney, N.S.W. Badly scalded about face and neck, October 1911.

SC 3—Female, born 1 a.m., 23.2.1871, London. In spring 1873 she fell into a bath of scalding water ; she eventually recovered. In taking her clothes off, the flesh of the left arm from elbow to armpit came away.

SC 4—Female, born 6.40 a.m., 20.3.1916, London. Placed, just after birth, on a bare stone hot-water bottle by nurse ; very severely burnt at back of thigh. This case is Example No. 19 on page 101.

SC 5—Male, born 11 p.m., approx., 5.4.1890, near London. Throat and mouth badly burnt at about 5 years through swallowing ammonia ; ill for months.

SC 6—Female, born 12.30 p.m., 24.1.1908, Philadelphia. In October 1912 went to hospital for 8 weeks, having suffered a severe scalding of the legs.

SC 7—Male, 3.23 a.m., 24.4.1928, Boston, Mass. Burnt by steam from radiator, 15.3.1931.

SC 10—Male, about 1 p.m., 23.8.1880, Jerseyville, Ill. Burnt leg with lye, through carelessness of nurse. See A.Q., March 1931, page 51.

An examination of these cases at once shows an area at the end of Virgo-Pisces and to a less extent at the end of the other mutable pair. These areas are marked in the two examples below ; and in the above 8 cases we have, successively :

SC 1. 25 ♐ rising
,, 2. ♂ 28 ♓ badly aspected
,, 3. ♀ 22 ♓
,, 4. ☉ 29 ♓
,, 5. . . . . . .
,, 6. ♄ 24 ♓
,, 7. ♄ 18½ ♐
,, 10. ♂ 21 ♍

Mars and Jupiter are commonly mutually involved, thus :

SC	1.	They are in sextile	
,,	2.	,, ,,	opposition, ♂ in ♓
,,	3.	······	······
,,	4.	,, ,,	trine
,,	5.	,, ,,	sextile, ♂ in ♐
,,	6.	,, ,,	trine
,,	7.	,, ,,	mutual reception, ♂ in ♓
,,	10.	,, ,,	♃ in ♈
Ex. No. 7.		,, ,,	conjunction, ♂ in ♓
Ex. No. 8.		,, ,,	square (wide) but ♂ in ♓ .

It is rather disconcerting to see so many technically good aspects between ♂ and ♃, but the facts are as above, and show that, though benefic aspects cannot, probably, in themselves cause or indicate accidents, yet, in combination with other factors, they may form a diathesis. [1]

[1] It is perhaps necessary to distinguish between what may be called the operative and the indicative elements in a horoscope. By astrological theory, every ill that can befall man does so only by reason of a definite malefic influence in his nativity. Thus, if a man has the Sun opposed to Mars, we know that certain disharmonies will inevitably enter his life, either interiorly or exteriorly, or both. This is an operative factor. But the very wide scope of the operative factor is narrowed down by what I call the indicative elements, which, in themselves often quite innocuous, will indicate the field in which the operative element will probably discharge. Sometimes the two factors are united in one configuration : for example, ☉ ☍ ♂ might fall in a definite area, and so the two elements would form a clear indication of specific trouble. Sometimes they are distinct, or at least as distinct as any parts of one map can be. When, therefore, in this book I may write as if a seemingly harmless factor had occasioned a grave evil, my intention rather is to convey the suggestion that the factor was indicative, but not operative (or causative, if we do not shy at this word in connection with astrology). I do not intend in any way to deny the proposition that every human misfortune must have a malefic factor in the natus corresponding to it.

Venus is commonly badly placed, usually being in some untoward relation with a fire-planet (Jupiter or Mars).

In every case except Nos. 7 and 10 there is an aspect between the Moon and Mars. In No. 7 she is square Uranus in Aries ; in 10, she is in ♈.

The striking proximity of the Sun and Mars which we observed in burns does not seem to occur in this category ; the Moon seems more significant. Saturn does not seem as common an afflictor as in burns, nor are the maps as a whole so conspicuous for mutable-sign afflictions.

It would certainly seem that scalding is a Piscean misfortune, for in the 11 cases I have used there are no less than 17 bodies in Pisces, omitting Uranus, Neptune, and Pluto, as being too slow of motion to be significant. The average would be 7. Mars is in Pisces 4 times. In 8 out of 11 cases he is in the sign of a benefic, a curious circumstance.

Scalds are also certainly connected with the signs Aries-Libra, for, counting as above, there are 29 bodies or points (asc. is included) in these signs, or twice the average.

Bodies in both Aries-Libra and Pisces therefore point to this danger.

Saturn is in Aries-Libra in 5 cases and when he is not in these signs he will be found to afflict a body therein.

Example No. 7

Boy, born 9.30 p.m., 11.4.1915, Epsom. Fell into bath of boiling water and died the same evening, 23.10.1920.

Circumstantial

There was no blame to be attached to the child. It would be difficult to say what rules baths, but there are two asphyxiation cases which involve the same article—the common factor seems to be about 25 ♊.

Example No. 7

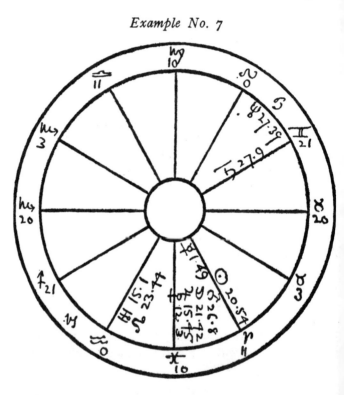

This map is eminently tragic, though it might be thought that the trines of Neptune would have prevented so shocking an end. Actually Moon-Neptune are " in stress."

Tables

Mercury is ill-placed in Aries and Jupiter in Pisces ; as regards houses, Neptune is weak in 9th.

There is a formidable array of bad stresses : ☉ ♄, ☽ ♅, ☽ ♆, ☿ ♂, ☿ ♄, ☿ ♆.

Directions

We find two powerful and sufficient directions : ☽ ☌ ♂ o-d and ♂ □ ♄ ($\frac{1}{4}°$).

Example No. 8

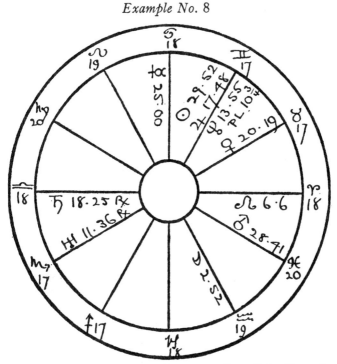

Male, born 12.57 p.m., June 21, 1894, Calcutta. At three weeks his fingers and toes were broken when his

nurse threw him, in self-defence, at a dog. At about
one year his feet were so badly scalded that he almost
died. At eight he nearly died of pneumonia. At twelve
he fell over a slope with his horse, which was killed ;
he broke his ribs. At fourteen he broke both arms at
roller-skating. On September 28, 1917, when inspect-
ing a train, he was caught between the footboard and
the platform and was rolled round and round ; almost
every bone was broken and his viscera crushed and
smashed, pelvis broken, and bladder injured. Constant operations as a result.

This is a sad history of accidents, but we take it here
as a case of scalding, due mainly, no doubt, like many
of the injuries, to Sun square Mars, in areas that we
have noted in this connection. Saturn is in an area of
falling, and Jupiter, most of all planets, seems evil in
17° ♊ – ♐ , as we shall see in subsequent sections.

Circumstantial

It would be difficult to find, in this map, specific indications of each misfortune, but it would probably be
by no means impossible to do this, if a detailed study
were made of the directions and if the student possessed
accurate knowledge of the many factors involved. But
such a task would be beyond the scope of this work.

It is clear that the major, the over-riding, influence
is Sun square Mars in mutables, but we must not over-
look Uranus on the cusp of the 2nd—bodies in this
position exercise a powerful influence upon the physical
welfare as well as the financial, by reason of the opposition to the cusp of the 8th. Certainly it is Uranus in
Scorpio in this position which indicates the damage to
the bladder, and, probably, the train-accident as a whole.

Tables

There are no weak sign- or house-positions, but there are some heavy stresses, i.e. ☉ ♅, ☉ ♆, ☽ ♆, ☿ ♄.

Directions

The arc for the railways accident is 23° 16′. This yields such important influences as ♄ ☌ ♅, ♀ ☌ ♆, ♃ △ ♅ [1] o-d.

By ¼° there are ♅ ⊼ ♃, ☉ □ Nodes.

When he was scalded at about one year, ♂ □ ☉ o-d would have been operative.

§ 9. GUNSHOTS

IN this connection we might expect to find significators of guns and shooting generally, and these might refer to a love of hunting, skill in taking aim, or marksmanship, a commercial occupation, such as the making of guns or ammunition, or to a purely fortuitous connection with guns, as when one is the victim of an accident without having any psychological interest in guns or shooting or hunting. Furthermore, it often happens that these categories overlap, yet they do not always do so.

Investigation is made difficult by one's ignorance of the facts of the cases or of the majority of them : for instance, Sebastian of Portugal (N.N. 576) was shot ; but whether he was interested in guns, and, if so, from what point of view, it would be hard to discover.

Not having many cases of accidental shooting, I have

[1] A benefic influence, but diminished by ♅ ⊼ ♃ ¼°.

been compelled to begin the examination of the subject with examples of intentional shooting, of which there is a number of authentic instances.

These seem to show, beyond dispute, that bullet-wounds, and probably all violent blows on small areas of the body, such as cuts and stabs, and some blows, are related to about 6° ♈-♎, there being some cases in which the same areas of ♋-♑ are involved.

Quoting a few cases from N.N.:

Archduke Franz Ferdinand	☽ 5 ♈
George of Greece	♂ 1 ♈, ♅ 6½ ♈
Don Carlos of Portugal	☉ 5 ♎, ♆ 5 ♈, ♂ 6 ♎
Louis Philippe of Portugal	♂ 8½ ♈
N.N. 332	♅ 6 ♎, ♄ 8 ♋
N.N.827 (first shot in Boer War)	Asc. 5 ♈
General Boulanger	Asc. 8½ ♋
Sebastian of Portugal	♃ 5 ♎ (ruler 4)
Grand Duchess Olga	♀ 7 ♎ (ruler 4)
Harry Thaw	♂ 8 ♎
N.N. 818	♃ 10 ♈ (ruler 4)
N.N.337	♄ 7½ ♈
N.N. 672	♄ 6 ♑, ♂ 8 ♎

These seem pretty conclusive. It will be also noted that these bodies show:

Many instances of bodies in the beginnings of the mutables.

Many at about 17° of the cardinals.

Many at about 16° of the mutables, especially ♊-♐.

This last area is connected with death by judicial sentence in P.A., but it is evident that it has a wider scope, for not all of the cases given above met their end in that manner, even though it might be considered that monarchs killed by anarchists have often been judged and condemned, in their absence and ignorance, by revolutionary " tribunals." This, however, could scarcely be said of suicides, [1] unless these people, as it were, judge and sentence themselves in the light of their own lives. Thus it seems a violent position, and this is apparently particularly true when Jupiter is there, as in Thaw's case and N.N. 672. In criminal maps it appears repeatedly, beyond all possibility of chance.

As for 17° cardinals, this is a notably violent area, in my experience.

There remains the beginnings of the mutables, from about 1° to 9°, but more often between 1° and 5°. This comes near to the notorious Aldebaran-Antares line, and it may be that their noxious properties, and in fact the peculiar values of all these areas, are connected with fixed stars. Certainly these mutable areas occur very frequently ; there is no need to labour to prove what will be sufficiently evident to anyone who troubles to study the class of horoscope with which we are dealing.

To differentiate the respective values of these three areas is, I confess, quite beyond my present powers ; they certainly indicate bloodshed.

None of these areas appears to have special reference to accidents as such ; and unfortunately I have not sufficient cases to enable me to decide what does indicate, in these gunshot cases, the element of accident. However, it is somewhat strange that in the 4 cases which I have there are Venus-Uranus afflictions in

[1] See note and cases in § 5. Suicides more often have afflictions in about 13° mutables.

each, including two conjunctions of these bodies.

Also 23° cardinals seems prominent.

Cases to study are :

N.N. 177 and 736 (Gambetta).

A lady, born 7 a.m., May 7, 1876, Illinois (ref. G 2). She was shot by accident in the neck by a boy, the bullet just missing the jugular vein. In this case the Taurus afflictions from Uranus in Leo are very characteristic ; and we also see two of the above four areas tenanted.

A fourth case is given below.

Example No. 9

Male, born 10.30 p.m., October 15, 1891, Lincolnshire. He was accidentally shot by a friend who had just bought a new gun, 3.30 p.m., 2.1.1930, and died about 8 p.m. of the same day.

Circumstantial

Does the negativity of this map, together with the strong ♎ element, point to suffering at the hands of others ? The map is a puzzle, and certainly does not seem to confirm my foregoing remarks, since the areas mentioned are hardly occupied. The nearest is the square in 9° ♊ ♓ .

Tables

Mars and Jupiter are in high-incidence signs, but nothing is ill-placed by house. There are two important stresses—☽ ♆ , and ☿ ♂ .

Directions

The arc is 38° 14′, By o-d the ascendant comes to the mutable cross, and so too Venus accompanied by

Uranus. The cusp of the 8th is opposed to its own ruler.

The $\frac{1}{4}°$ measure brings the Sun to Uranus, and, it is interesting to note, also brings Mars to the 6° ♎ area.

Example No. 9

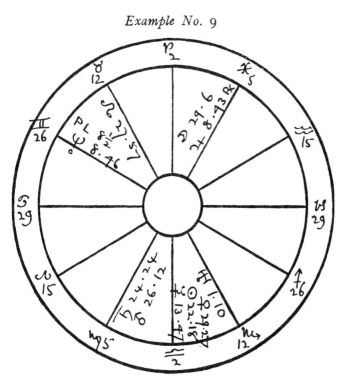

§ 10. BLOWS

WE now come to some categories of accident that are extremely wide and ill-defined. I have named the present class as above, for lack of a better appellation.

But blows are obviously of many kinds. A bullet strikes a blow, so does a fist and even a vehicle. The various forms of crushing that I have placed in the next section are not very different. Even a wound from a shell might be classed as a blow, and a fall is really a blow from the ground or whatever other object is struck in falling.

However, I have tried to use the word blow fairly strictly, and have placed crushing in a separate section and also wounds and falls. Under " Vehicular Accidents " I have placed only those in which the victim was himself passenger or driver. When he is struck or crushed by a vehicle, the case is placed under the appropriate section. Strictly, " Blows " includes no case where blood is shed—such are placed under Wounds.

The reader must therefore take these groupings as being the best that I could do by way of classifying. And, where classification is so difficult, one must not expect to find very precise horoscopic *differentiæ*.

Cases for study :

BL 1—Male, 1 a.m., 16.2.1888, Manchester. Right eye burst by a golf-ball in playing with a friend.

BL 2—Female, about 4 p.m., 19.4.1902, Erith, Kent. Left leg lost below hip as a result of blow, 17.9.1920.

BL 3—Male, 10.38 p.m., 4.3.1918, Melksham, Wilts. Ran in front of lorry 23.10.1924 ; knee-cap smashed and back of head damaged.

BL 4—Female, 2 a.m., 21.2.1899, London. Left leg amputated at eleven years by reason of a blow received in play.

BL 5—Male, 5.5 a.m., 8.9.1893, Bromham, Wilts. Load slipped from a crane hook and badly knocked the back of his hand, fracturing several small bones.

BL 6—Male, 6.30 p.m., 4.2.1877, Wrexham, Denbigh. Cracked jaw in starting up a lorry—the handle flew back. Early 1926.

BL 7—Male, 10 a.m., 12.10.1895, London. Smashed leg in lorry accident at Baghdad, about end 1919. Leg now shorter than the other.

BL 8—Male, born 1 a.m., 26.7.1920, Sydney, N.S.W. Killed by car, 29.6.1927.

BL 9—Male, born 4.50 p.m., 11.2.1871, Sydney, N.S.W. Run down in August 1923 by a car and legs fractured. In December 1922 building material fell on his head and he sustained a bad wound.

BL 14—Female, born 3.40 p.m., 11.9.1922, Boston, Mass. Killed by auto, 5.10.1929.

BL 17—Male, born 11.53 p.m., July 6, 1908, Stuttgart. From *Sterne und Mensch*, November 1931. Native was hurt internally while boxing, and as a result of X-ray treatment his spleen was burnt, so that he is not expected to survive his twenty-eighth year. An extraordinary natus, with which compare RL 3 on page 107.

BL 18—Female, born 5.15 p.m., November 19, 1879, Midlands. Knocked down by a car 11.1.1930, and her pelvis fractured. Fully recovered.

BL 19—Female, born 11 p.m., April 13, 1901, London. Hit in face by lorry and knocked over. Had to have leg amputated below knee ; then, because of sepsis, had to have knee removed as well.

N.N. 853, 890, Nos. 3 and 4 in S.D.

Two Exx. below.

In testing these and other cases for typical areas, I find the following worth mentioning :

1. 4°–8° Aries-Libra : The essence of this area seems to be effusion of blood, and it hardly occurs in these blows cases (20 in all) except where blood is shed, as in BL 9 above and Ex. 10 below. It occurs only 4 times in the 20, and therefore seems to have no specific relation to this class of case.

2. 15°–19° cardinals: This area occurs 10 times, with strict observation of the limits of the area ; it may therefore be considered important. I am inclined to suggest that the essence of this place is falling (with which we deal later), but it may have a much wider significance.[1]

3. 20°–24° cardinals : This occurs 9 times, but I cannot suggest what its specific value may be.

4. 24°–28° fixed : This area, which has not occurred in the previous types of accident, appears 14 times, and must be considered important in this class of mis-chance.

5. 0°–9° mutables : This appears 14 times, but is, of course, more than twice the extension of the other areas.

6. 15°–19° mutables : This has also been noted be-fore, and now occurs 13 times, so that, with 24°–28° fixed, it is really the principal area in these cases.

One may anticipate criticism by admitting that these areas cover in all 116°, or about a third of the zodiac,

[1] It is interesting to observe here, *en passant*, that Mrs. Bessie Leo and the present writer both have Saturn square the asc. in almost the same areas (17°♋︎ ♎︎), and that both had dangerous falls in childhood (♋︎). See *Esoteric Astrology*, " A Human Document." The author's fall was caused by his propelling a perambulator, in which he was, or should have been, reclining, until it went, with him inside it, to the bottom of a sandpit. Nor did he altogether escape danger of crushing, for a very corpulent grandparent, arriving at the house after a hot walk, all but sat down heavily upon him. This probably has something to do with ♅ in 1st (1st=grandparents).

so that it would be strange if some planet did not appear in one or two of them in any case. What we usually find, however, in accident horoscopes, is a *severe affliction* involving these areas, or some of them. Again, it must be remembered that accidents are not rare things, and, just as these areas are frequently occupied, so human beings often meet with accidents ; it is probably rather exceptional to meet with a man who has never met with any physical mishap, though of course in this work we are concerned, as far as possible, with serious ones.

Turning to characteristic aspects in cases such as these, it is rare to find a bad case in which one of the three hylegiacals (☉, ☽, asc.) or the ruler is not in major bad aspect with ♂ or ♅, ♄ afflictions being rare in this group.

I now take two examples, of which the former affords an interesting comparison with Example No. 8.

Example No. 10

Lady, born 5 a.m., May 5, 1905, Pasadena, California. On March 1, 1925, she was dragged 30 feet under a car which had struck her ; she was terribly wounded ; her arms were slashed, her backbone dislocated, causing some paralysis, her facial bones were badly crushed, her sternum was broken ; she was nine months in hospital with two trained nurses.

This is a case of mixed conditions, and might equally well be placed under three or four sections.

Circumstantial

The Sun and the ruler of the 8th receive the full force of the opposition of Mars, in angles and forming. The

Moon moves to the square of Saturn, showing, probably, the fractured bones. Mercury and Venus, though they have good aspects, are separating from them by retrograde motion. Of the 6 areas, the 1st, 4th, and

Example No. 10

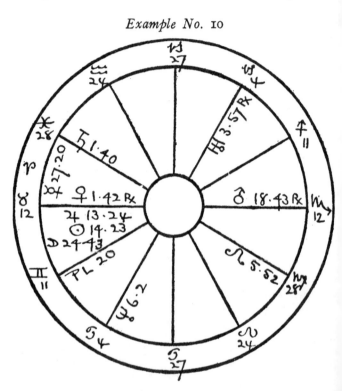

5th are well marked. Cars, as such, I place under Jupiter and the 9th, and it will be seen that planet and house are heavily involved. Note the effusion of blood (arms slashed) and the involvement of Area 1, which I connect with bloodshed, or at least the breaking of

the skin. ☽ ☐ ♄ ⚹ seems to show the arms; back-bone and sternum come under the ♉ ♍ afflictions, and the face under the afflicted bodies in the 1st house and the cardinal opposition. For paralysis, see E.P.A., but the aspects between the significant planets are good—hence the condition was not permanent, and would not have occurred at all had the rest of the map not been so violent. Here, as often, the indicative factors are in themselves harmless, but point the direction for the action of the operative elements.

Tables

Sun, Mercury, and Saturn are in unfavourable signs, and Mercury and Saturn in unfavourable houses. The bad stresses are ☉ ♅ , ☽ ♄ , ♂ ♅ —characteristic and powerful.

Directions

The arc is 19° 50'. The directions are singularly striking, and offer a crushing reply to those who reject and asperse symbolic measures. By o-d we have asc. ☐ ♄ , ☿ ☍ ♂ , ☉ ♃ ☌ ♅ and ♂ to cusp 8th, whilst good nursing is shown by ♆ ⚹ ☽ . By ¼° we have the following formidable progressions— ☉ ♃ ☍ ♂ , ☽ ☐ ♄ (applying).

Example No. 11

Male, born 2.2 p.m., June 17, 1890, near London. A naval pensioner who was aboard ship, when, coming on deck in response to a call from his wife, his head was struck as he stood before her by the tackle of a crane, so that he was instantly decapitated.

Psychological

An interesting point may be touched on here. Does

the natus only relate to consciousness? Here it is
probable that there was no pain and no consciousness
of what happened. The map is not violently afflicted,
and even the addition (by those who believe in them)

Example No. 11

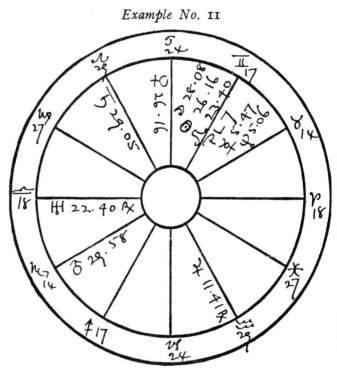

of such positions as Mars heliocentric (in 18° ♐) and
Saturn heliocentric (4° ♍) does not make the map as
violent as a purely factual view of the nativity would
require. The reaction points do not altogether solve
the problem, either.

However, I incline myself to a factual view of the

horoscope ; that is to say, I believe that it shows things apart from their reaction in the consciousness. A man struck dead instantaneously would have appropriate directions and natal afflictions.

Circumstantial

The action of the wife appears through Venus and Libra ; the fact that he was aboard for the purpose of drawing back-pay is indicated by Mars in the 2nd ; Neptune in 8th points to an end near the sea ; Uranus, conjunction ascendant, must be held responsible for the blow to the head.

Of our areas, 2, 3, 4, and 5 are involved, though 4 is only to be included by an extension of the orbs.

The worst position is probably Uranus on asc., square ruler 8th, and with three sesquiquadrates from that house.

Tables

Mars is in an unfavourable sign, and Saturn and Uranus in bad houses. Stresses are— ☉ ♄ , ☉ ♅ , ☿ ♄ , ☿ ♅ .

Directions

Unfortunately, the date of death is not known.

§ 11. CRUSHING

UNDER this term I include certain cases of collision where the victim has been described as crushed rather than cut or fractured ; and there are also cases that are more precisely described as crushing, wherein weights have fallen on the native.

Cases to Study

Two are given below as examples.

N.N. 390.

CR 1—Female, born 10.30 a.m., 13.4.1899, Geneva. Crushed by a car, 2.50 p.m., 28.1.1909.

CR 2—Female, born 1 p.m., 2.5.1905, Geneva. Crushed by a car, 11.50 a.m., 14.8.1906.

CR 3—Male, born 3.40 p.m., 10.8.1907, Geneva ; died 10.50 a.m., 12.12.1910. Crushed by a tram.

CR 4—Male, 2 a.m., 8.12.1884, Devonshire, foot crushed as child by a dropped brick.

CR 5—Male, born 11.30 p.m., 1.10.1882, London ; severely crushed a leg and damaged right knee by fall of a heavy weight, 11.30 a.m., 14.3.1929.

CR 6—Male, born 11.12 a.m., 14.12.1885, 51° 26' N., 2° 10' W. Thrown from pony between four and five years ; bone in foot broken by horse at nine years ; nearly drowned at twelve ; crushed in collapse of football stand, when many were killed, April 1901 ; finger severely cut when mowing grass.

Regarding this last case we may say that the accidents from horses (see also Section 19) may be ascribed to the ♂ – ♃ – ♄ configuration (♂ is only in aspect with ♃ and ♄ by minor aspect—perhaps ♅ here usurps his part, as is often the case), and also to ☉ ☌ ♆, which also may be the cause of the escape from drowning. It is fortunate that ☽ ☍ ♂ is separating.

In regard to the first three of the above cases and N.N. 390, all of which concern vehicles and collisions, I do not think that it is without significance that in each of them Neptune is afflicted by an opposition. One may be inclined to place motor-cars under Jupiter ; and Neptune, though he is often related to this planet through Pisces, is not as a rule connected by astrologers with Sagittarius. This, however, may be a mistake. It is possible that Neptune " understudies " both positive and negative Jupiter. In mythology he is said to have created horses, and is usually represented in a chariot. Jupiter is not abnormally afflicted in these cases, nor, indeed, Mercury.

The principal afflictions in these four are respectively,

CR 1. ☉ □ ♂, ☽ ☍ ♅, ♄ ☍ ♆.
CR 2. ☉ ♃ ☍ ♂, ♅ ☍ ♆.
CR 3. (♂ ☌ ♅) ☍ ♆.
N.N. 390. (☉ ☌ ♀) ☍ ♆, ☽ ☍ ♄, asc. ☍ ☿.

The area which appears consistently is the beginning of the mutables.

In CR 4 there is a powerful ☉ ☍ ♄, and it is noteworthy that in this case the weight fell from above, and the crushing did not result from a lateral blow in the horizontal plane, as is to some extent the case in most vehicular accidents. Saturn afflicts from above in the horoscope. The Sun is in a dangerous area, and the Moon and Jupiter, though strong, are in another. Mercury and Mars receive the square of Uranus, but the trine of Moon-Jupiter. The native, though lame, is a man of brilliant parts and an exceptionally able debater, as well as a keen motor-cyclist.

In CR 5 we see that Saturn once again afflicts from above. The Moon has the square of Uranus, and there is Mercury conjunction Mars. Another keen debater and writer on economics. Critical areas are hardly represented, unless we allow Sun 9° ♎. The injury was temporary, though acutely painful.

Both these cases—in fact, all seven—show afflictions to hylegiacals.

Example No. 12

Male, born 1 a.m., 8.6.1891, Geneva.   Crushed by a motor, 8.45 p.m., 30.8.1920.

Circumstantial

If we are right in suggesting a connection between Neptune and automobiles, we certainly find some confirmation here, for Neptune, in the 3rd, is the weak planet, having a close conjunction of Pluto and the square of Saturn.   Jupiter rising, and in its own sign, should have been a preservative according to traditional astrology, despite the bad aspects which it receives (as also good ones). But Table III has shown the weakness of Jupiter-Pisces. The ☉ □ ♃ is, of course, exactly in critical degrees. As a powerful malefic aspect to a hylegiacal we have ☽ ☌ ♂. To this, certainly, must the fatal result of the accident be ascribed ; there is nothing else that is really violent.

Tables

Jupiter is weak by sign and the Sun and Saturn by house.

There are strong unfavourable stresses— ☉ ♂, ☉ ♅, ☉ ♆, ♂ ♅, ♂ ♆.

Directions

By o–d, ☉ △ ♃ asc. (from □).

By 4/7ths, ♃, asc. □ ☽ ♂, ♀ ☌ ♆ PL, ☉ ☌ ☽ ♂.

By ¼°, ♄ 8 ♃, □ ☉.

Example No. 13

Male, born 3.55 a.m., 16.1.1876, Chilcompton, 51° 16′ N. and 2½° W.

In 1924 a 1 cwt. bundle fell from a crane on to the top of his head, causing temporary total paralysis and congested liver ; no bones were broken.

Circumstantial

In this horoscope, as in the foregoing, we find a failure of a rising Jupiter to protect, unless we assume that without it the accident would have had a worse result, as, indeed, is possible but insusceptible of proof. But Jupiter is afflicted. As in CR 5 and 6 above, Saturn afflicts, but he is low in the map, though above Venus, ruler of 6th. Note ☉ ☿ □ ♅ for paralysis (E.P.A. Paralysis). Also the afflictions to Jupiter, and Mars in 29½° ♓, for liver. Case SC 4, with ☉ in exactly the same spot, suffered from jaundice ; see also Ex. No. 9.

This is a really badly afflicted map.

Example No. 13

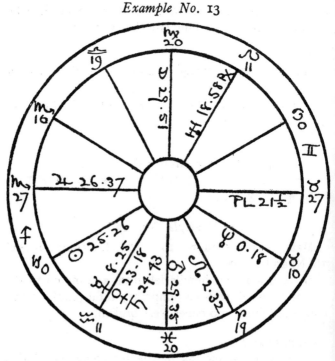

As regards areas, see ♀ ♄ in and near 25° fixed, mentioned under " Blows." The two mutable areas do not appear.

Tables

This case is not one that supports the value of the

tables, for Mercury in 3rd is the only weak house-position, and there are none by sign. Also there is but one stress— ♂ ♆ .

Directions
   ⅛° PL ☍ asc., ♅ ☍ ♄ . ¼° ♃ ⚹ ☿ .
   4/7th ♆ ☍ asc. ; o–d ☽– ♂ □ ♅ .

These are ample and characteristic. The good direction ♃ ⚹ ☿ is sufficient to mitigate the consequences of the accident to some extent, but it must be borne in mind that the natus itself is an unpromising one.

§ 12. WOUNDS AND CUTS

IN this section I propose to deal with cases of which the principal characteristic is the effusion of blood, as distinct from the application of force, as in crushing and blows. Here, as in gunshots, it is easier to obtain cases of non-accidental injury than of accidental.

We may, for instance, quote the Empress Elizabeth of Austria, N.N. 809, who was stabbed to death by an anarchist. This shows the malefic influence in the beginnings of the mutables (♅ 5° ♓) that we have so often seen, and also 17° cardinals (♂ 17° ♑). The actual danger seems principally shown by ☽ ☌ ♄ , involving another area already mentioned.

It has been observed that probably the area at the beginning of the cardinals (and chiefly ♈ ♎) is connected with cuts and loss of blood, but in the Empress's case we have only ☉ 3° ♑ , barely within orbs of Mars.

Cases to study are :

W 1—Male, born 2.45 a.m., 13.12.1878, 51° 9′ N., 53′ E. Cut an artery, 25.1.1914.

W 2—Male, born 9.20–9.30 a.m., 23.6.1917, Meerut, India, 29° N., 78° E. Broke collar-bone at gymnastics, 16.7.1930 ; badly cut hands by breaking bottle, and also stung by wasp, 3.9.1930.

W 3—Male, 5 a.m., 12.1.1915, Buenos Aires. Was destined for the Argentine Navy, but age of twelve cut off a finger in playing with an axe.

W 4—Male, born about 4 a.m., 15.12.1879, New York. Leaned his hand against a mirror, which fell, cutting his foot severely.

N.N. 832, forehead badly cut by glass, which had been broken by a fall of snow. I suspect snow and ice of coming chiefly under ♆, which in this case is in 25° ♈.

Case from B.J.A., May 1921, sex not recorded, 4.45 a.m., 17.7.1904, Glasgow. Died February 1907, having swallowed a knitting-needle which penetrated the throat.

In all of these the beginnings of the mutables are occupied, with the exception of the curious and not easily paralleled knitting-needle case. There is also a tendency for the last decan of ♊ ♐ to be occupied— No. 2 is the only exception to this, which, generally, I have connected with drowning.[1] The middle of the cardinals is well represented : No. 1, nil ; No. 2, ♀ 17° ♋ ; No. 3, ♂ 16° ♑ ; No. 4, ☽ 19° ♑ ; N.N. 832, ♄ 15° ♑.

Three cases in this class show a body in 24° ♒, and in another we have ♂ ☍ PL *circa* 24° ♉. W. 4 has

[1] Many cases of drowning involve the vessel receiving a blow or " stab."

PL 26° ♉, so that the knitting-needle case alone
escapes this category, which horoscope, from the
standpoint of traditional astrology, we should have
expected to show a fixed affliction, owing to the local-
isation of the wound.

Example No. 14

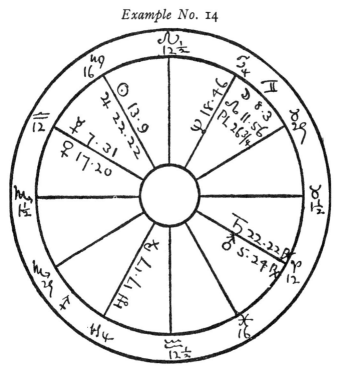

This is a mixed case, being partly of the nature of a
blow.

Girl, born 10 a.m., September 6, 1909, London.
When she reached her fourteenth birthday she asked
to be allowed to go alone to a fair. She was struck in

the mouth by a swing-boat and rendered unconscious. Her upper lip and tongue were split.

Psychological

The slight degree of self-will which went with this accident is in accord with the Martian ascendant and ruler in Aries.

The native had no recollection of what happened, and this seems to agree with the befogging effects of Neptune, afflicting so many bodies so severely from a mental house. She seems to have strayed absent-mindedly within range of the boat.

Circumstantial

We have a strong evidence of accidents in the areas— Uranus afflicted in 17° cardinals, Mars-Mercury in the beginnings of Aries-Libra, and the Sun in 13° Virgo, not far from the 17° mutables area.

The lights are well-placed, hence the absence of grave after-effects. There was no severe permanent disfigurement.

Localisation

The whole of this branch of our inquiry will be treated of later, but we may certainly relate the tongue and lip to Mercury, opposed to Mars, but fortunately separating. This last fact may account for the healing of the wound and removal of disfigurement.

Tables

Mercury and Saturn are weak by house. The stresses are ⊙ ♅, ⊙ ♆, ☿ ♅.

Directions

At 14 we find ⊙ □ PL, ☿ ☍ ♄, ♅ □ Asc., ♂ □ ♆, ☽ □ ♃, all o-d—a most formidable array.

§ 13. VEHICULAR ACCIDENTS

UNDER this head are classed accidents wherein the native was himself driving a car or motor-cycle, or riding a bicycle, or was a passenger. Cases of persons driving carts, traps, and other horse-drawn vehicles are in these days rather rare. In cases wherein the native is a pedestrian, struck or crushed by a vehicle, I have classed the horoscope under another head, as has been explained. Such classifications must necessarily be very unsatisfactory, but they are perhaps as good as can be found for practical purposes, especially in a work that does not pretend to be exhaustive, but only introductory.

Accidents of this kind conform well to traditional rules. As might be expected, afflictions to the mutable planets, Mercury and Jupiter, are almost always present, the former body being more in evidence in cycling accidents, and perhaps in accidents arising on the course of routine journeys, such as to and from employment. Jovian travels usually have the exploratory element. Saturn afflictions tend to broken bones, Uranus to shock. Afflictions in mutables, and especially in Gemini-Sagittarius, are common, and so too are afflictions from the 3rd to the 9th. Many areas which we have already noticed will be found to appear, but sporadically ; and until their intrinsic meanings have been discovered it seems impossible to try to trace their values in individual cases.

Cases for Study

V 1—Male, born 3 a.m., 21.4.1896, Grantham, Lincs. Thigh broken 28.8.1901, right arm broken 27.9.1905, and amputated four days later. Thrown from motor-cycle by collision with car ; shoulders, knee and face badly cut, 6.9.1927. Thrown from motor-cycle by skid on leaves ; shoulder, thigh, and leg badly cut, 21.10.1928. Note that all accidents happened in autumn.

V 2—Male, born 8.57 p.m., 25.10.1904, London. Killed when motoring to see the total eclipse of 29.6.1927 in 6° ♋.

V 3—Male, 1 a.m. 15.1.1885, Aldershot, Hants. Bad cycling accident, killed later in Macedonia.

V 4—Male, between 10 and 11 a.m., 13.5.1903, Richmond, Yorks. Accident when motor-cycling, concussion and forehead badly scarred, 17.1.1931.

V 5—Male, 11 p.m., 19.11.1867, Frome, Somerset. Serious cycling accident, 19.12.1913 ; run into by girl and now limps.

V 6—Male, 6.45 a.m., 3.12.1895, about 17° 30' N., 72° 30' E. Broke ankle during night of 28.5.1927, in long-distance motor-bike race in Wales, and hurt thigh.

V 7—Male, 7.05 a.m., 29.2.1904, Devizes, Wilts. Ran into steam-roller when on motor-cycle going to work on morning of 20.6.1921. Leg broken in several places. Cp. V 24, below (same day).

V 15—Male, 7.30–7.45 p.m., 9.8.1897, Melksham, Wilts. Broke leg in motor-cycle accident, 17.8.1928; leg badly set, had to be rebroken and reset.

V 21—Female, 11 a.m., 1.5.1878, Hastings. Badly crushed by fall under cart when cycling. Hearing on one side destroyed.

V 22—Male, 9.0 p.m., 31.10.1901, Nanticoke, Pa. Severely cut about chin and head in car-collision with astrologer born under ♒.

V 23—Male, 2 a.m., 7.3.1907, Pennsylvania. Killed 20.11.1921, when riding bike ; hit by car and thrown under wheels. A twin-sister suffered from goitre.

V 24—Female, about lunch-time, 29.2.1904, London. Run over by cart outside home (afflictions involve ♋) and right leg amputated at knee, January 1908. See V 7 above.

N.N. 893, 979.

Three examples below.

I have used in all 21 cases in this category, others arriving after the work had been done. Typical contacts are : ♃ in affliction with ♂ , ♄ or ♅ ; ♃ □ ☿ ; ☿ in affliction with ♂ or ♅ ; ♂ in affliction with ♅.

Skids are probably Uranian, accidents in fogs Neptunian or possibly Plutonic, though one would probably do well to guard against collisions with drainage works in the road when under the malevolent action of this body.

Mars occurs 5 times in Virgo in these 21 cases, but why he should seem to have this affinity in such accidents I do not know. He is only once in Gemini and not at all in Libra ; other signs are average.

Example No. 15

Male, born at Ipswich, 11.48 a.m., November 3, 1911. Died when pillion-riding from his job with a fellow-workman. They were knocked down by a car and the native's head was terribly injured. Accident was at 5.45 p.m., October 10, 1931, at Nottingham. Died next day.

Psychological

The tables show that Capricorn-rising is rarely

Example No. 15

involved in any accidents, and in this case we may
observe that the victim was in no way responsible.

Circumstantial

This map came to hand after the earlier part of the
section had been written, but it agrees well with what
had been stated, despite the brilliantly good aspects
that also occur in the natus. It is curious that the Sun
is fairly free from affliction, the opposition to Saturn
being wide. The square of Pluto to the Moon implies
that the former can be very evil.

Tables

There are no bad sign-positions, which is additional evidence of lack of psychological responsibility on the part of the native. By house Uranus and Neptune are weak.

There are no evil stresses. This case seems, in fact, to be one in which the chief responsibility lies with Pluto, and this planet was not embodied in Table III.

Directions

The age was just twenty. By one-degree Mars is square radical Moon, exact, and asc. in conj. Uranus. By ¼°, together with some apparently good directions, there is Saturn opp. Jupiter. Note also that Uranus is getting near the square of Mercury-Saturn by o-d. By primary direction the asc. is opp. Pluto *cum latitudine*—latitude being a very important item in regard to this planet.

Example No. 16

Lad born in Hertfordshire about 10.50 p.m., August 2, 1912. Intelligent, handsome, and a fine character. Coming home March 25, 1930, on a newly-bought motor-bicycle, he ran into a lorry and was killed instantaneously.

Circumstantial

Here also the Sun has only a wide opposition, whilst both it and the Moon receive good rays from a strong Jupiter, ruling 8th. But this planet is again opposed to Saturn, and Mercury is with Mars and in square to the two others. Once again the Moon is square Pluto, though dissociate.

Example No. 16

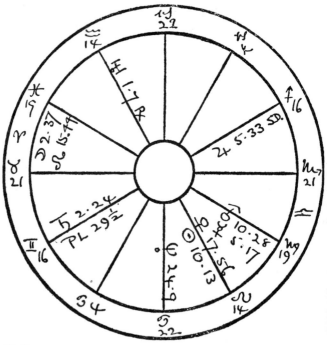

Tables

Mars in Virgo is the only bad sign- or house-position.

Bad stresses are : ☉ ♄, ☉ ♅, ☿ ♂.

Directions

The arc = 17° 39′. There are no close 1° or ¼°
directions, though there are many within a year or so
among the scattered mutable bodies. The ascendant,
it seems to me, should probably be about 22½° ♉ ; we
should then have asc. □ ♂ 1°, ☌ ♄ 4/7ths, and ruler
□ asc. ¼°.

Speaking from the standpoint of traditional astrology, I should not have expected early death either in this case or in the preceding ; but it is evident that Pluto must be taken into serious account in such maps, and his afflictions to Luna, in particular, seem dangerous.

Those interested in hypotheticals may care to observe that in all three of the examples given in this section, *Isis* is a potent afflictor. In No. 15 she is opp. Moon, Moon, sq. asc. ; in No. 16 she is conj. Moon ; in No. 17 she is on the asc., conj. ruler and Sun. I have always regarded her action as like that of a violent Mercury, or perhaps like Mercury + Mars.

Example No. 17

Lad born 6.30 a.m., September 21, 1907, Melksham, Wilts. He was killed when cycling, by reason of a skid which threw him in front of a bus. He died almost instantaneously, no bones were broken, but the liver was ruptured. Accident was at 6.25 p.m., December 8, 1926.

Circumstantial

Not a difficult case for which to account. There are heavy mutable afflictions which again involve Pluto ; and there are likewise cardinal afflictions of a serious character. The comparative strength of Jupiter is the most noteworthy feature of the horoscope on the good side, but Jupiter has three minor bad aspects. Note that this was a push-bicycle accident, and observe the prominence of Mercury.

Tables

Saturn is weak both by sign and by house—note that

Example No. 17

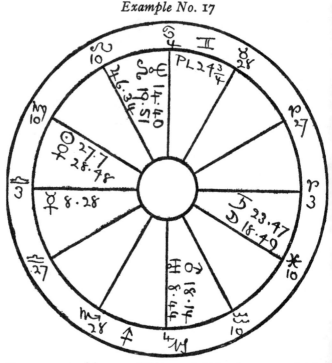

it was a crushing accident, and this planet would be expected to figure malefically.

Stresses are also heavily Saturnian, with one Uranian, for the skid: ☽ ♄, ☿ ♅, ♂ ♄.

Directions

Arc 19° 13'. By 1° the chief feature is the passage of the mutables ♄, PL, ☉, ♀ to affliction with the cardinals ♂ and ♅. These form various evil aspects around the time, some very close, e.g. ruler and lady 8th □ ♂ in 4th. ♂ comes near 8 ♃, and ☽ □ ☿ ♅.

♅ is △ ☉ ♀, but carries too serious afflictions to be of use. There are severe and characteristic ¼° directions ; ☽ ♂ ♄ is very near to time.

§ 14. FALLS

OF these I have used 31 well-defined cases. The chief index seems to be afflictions between Cancer and Libra, and, not quite so frequently, between these and Capricorn. Aries does not appear to be in general a sign of falling. Saturn is in Cancer in no less than 6 cases, and, in the two Jovian signs, 4 times each, so that these three sign-positions cover almost half the cases. When Saturn is not in Cancer it will often be found that one of the other malefics is therein : Cancer is undoubtedly connected with falls, as Capricorn is traditionally the sign of rising and climbing. But the commonest ascendants are Leo (7) and Virgo (6).

As regards the location of bodies in signs generally, I find, taking the rising sign and the signs occupied by the eight more quickly moving bodies, that the first three contain only 44 points, against an average of 70, Gemini being lowest. Leo, Libra, and Scorpio occur most often.

The four most commonly occupied areas are the first few degrees of the cardinals and of the mutables, and about 18° cardinals and 14°-17° mutables. These areas have been mentioned before in Section 11, " Blows "—falls involve a blow.

The map of the Prince of Wales,[1] who has had some severe falls in the hunting-field, illustrates all four of these areas.

[1] The present Duke of Windsor.

Cases to Study

F 1—Male, born 7.10 p.m., 12.4.1865, Yorks. On 14.10.1883 he fell from a mast at sea and broke his back and leg.

F 2—Male, born 12.30 a.m., 16.8.1891, 51° 26′ N., 2° 12′ W. Broke leg and arm in falling off a girder when avoiding a truss that slipped when being hoisted. This occurred in South Africa, February-March 1925.

F 3—Male, 12.43 a.m., 7.11.1922, 51° 24′ N., 2° 10′ W. Fractured arm in falling off a seesaw, 16.7.1930.

F 4—Female, born 11.45 p.m., 31.10.1886, London. Paralysed at age four through fall from swing.

F 5—Female, born 4 a.m., 1.9.1898, Melksham, Wilts. Fell on landing-stage when getting into a boat and badly bruised base of spine. An abscess grew, March 1915, and this recurred January 1919, and February 1924.

F 6—Female, born 6.24 p.m., 21.2.1875, London. At age seven fell at children's party and injured right hip. On back for five years and sustained a shortening of the right leg. On 14.6.1910 fell and injured pelvis, an abscess appeared, and right leg was removed at hip.

F 7—Female, 1.12 p.m., 1.6.1890, London. At age of three-and-a-half she fell and broke her collar-bone, causing a permanent injury to the spine and general paralysis ; at ten she had an operation, which was a complete failure and left her a cripple.

F 8—Female, born 1.10 a.m., 15.11.1914, Brentwood, Essex. Had a severe fall at seaside when on holiday in fall of 1925. Spinal abscess developed, and she was on her back for three years. An interesting instance of the use of the reaction points.

F 9—Male, born 11.45 p.m., 6.10.1890, Melksham, Wilts. Operation to knee for varicose veins, September 1914. In March 1915 water on knee developed as a result of a fall, injuring the operated knee.

F 12—Female, 7.30 a.m., 23.11.1867, New York City. On 19.8.1929, tripped on doorstep and fell, hurting left leg and foot, fracturing left arm, and cutting head.

F 13—Female, 7.11 p.m., 6.8.1884, London. Slipped and dislocated right foot at tarsal junction of the metatarsal arch ; no pain and complete cure, contrary to expectations. About 1 p.m., 16.11.1923.

F 14—Male, 10.45 a.m., 23.4.1918, Melksham, Wilts. Fell off box and cut back of head very badly, June 1922.

F 15—Female, 5.20 a.m., 14.3.1898, Greenwich, Kent. Broke arm at two years ; legs broken at ten by surgical operation to rectify deformity.

F 17—Male, 8.30 p.m., 9.4.1877, Sydney, N.S.W. At five years fell and split his head open on stone curb.

F 19—Male (?), 8 a.m., 26.8.1907, London. Creeping paralysis as a result of fall from a bicycle, October 1924.

F 26—Female, about 1.15 a.m., 6.7.1887, Parkstone, Dorset. Broke collar-bone as a child.

F 27—Male, 5.34 a.m., 5.1.1882, London. Has been unable to walk since childhood, owing to an injury to the spine caused by a child having withdrawn his chair.

F 28—Admiral Byrd (see A.Q., June 1930), 11.30 a.m., 25.10.1888, Winchester, Virginia.

F 31—Male, 2 a.m., 16.10.1868, Manchester ; ref. M.A., January 1917. Thrown from horse and right arm broken ; thigh pierced by spiked railings.

F 33—Child, born 7 p.m., 2.2.1925, Bremen. Fell from window, shattering skull, 8.8.1930. *Sterne und Mensch*, December 1931.

Other cases :

King William III was thrown from his horse, and died in consequence.

N.N. 157, 252, 802, 976.

Example No. 18

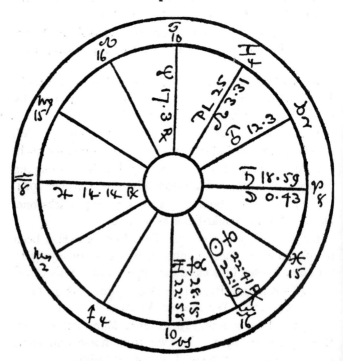

Map of the younger of male twins, born 9 and 9.30
p.m. February 12, 1910, Melksham, Wilts. The
younger, whose map appears above, is mentally
deficient as the result of a fall from his perambulator at
the age of two. He struck his brother violently on the
head on another occasion, but without serious result.

Circumstantial

There are no planets in mutable signs, but the
cardinal areas are well represented. As regards the
unfortunate reaction on the mind, Jupiter, ruling 3rd,
is badly involved, and Saturn in Aries receives the
square of the elevated Neptune.

Tables

These do not throw much light on this case. There
are, however, three stresses of a characteristic kind—
☿ ♄, ♂ ♅, ♂ ♆.

Directions

By one-degree progression several aspects are close—
♂ catches up to ⊼ ♃, ♃ to □ ♆, ♆ to □ ♄.

Example No. 19

Girl, born 6.40 a.m., March 20, 1916, London. This is
Case SC 4, and the same map has figured in the never-
ending controversies regarding the pre-natal epoch,
as well as being quoted under " Jaundice " in E.P.A.
The child had a severe fall 16.8.1926, when on holiday
in the Isle of Wight. She was playing on the roof of
an outhouse, stepped back, fell through a skylight, and

Example No. 19

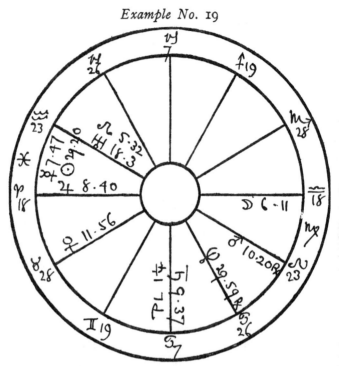

was found unconscious, on a heap of glass, having fallen about thirteen feet on to stone steps, which just missed the spine. She was uncut, and there were no lasting ill-effects. The author's daughter, and first cousin of F 8 above.

Psychological

We have said that Aries is not a sign of falling. But one cannot fall without first in some manner climbing. and Aries, especially with a rising Jupiter, is certainly fond of mounting upwards. It is a somewhat reckless map.

Circumstantial

The two cardinal areas, and one of the mutables, are represented, and ☽ ☐ ♄ points clearly to a fall ; it is applying ; but perhaps the mutual reception saved the native from the worst result. Again, Moon and Jupiter are in elevation over Saturn. Mars in 5th shows danger on holiday, but the trine of Jupiter is naturally protective.

Tables

Mercury is weak by house. There are some marked stresses, bringing out the action of Saturn : ☉ ♄ , ☽ ♄ , ☽ ♅ , ☿ ♄ , ♄ ♅ .

Directions

Sun square Saturn and Neptune conj. Mars amply explain this mischance. By ¼° we have, happily, only ☽ ☍ ♃ and M.C. ☍ ♄ .

§ 15. MACHINERY

ANY accident that results from, or in any way involves, an instrument artificially made of metal, might, I think, be placed in this section. Utensils as a class probably come under Mercury, and, more particularly, under Virgo. But this section treats of accidents with machinery so designated in a more precise manner. A number of the cases already listed have in some measure involved machines ; most vehicular accidents certainly do so.

I have very few cases that in the more restricted sense are concerned with instruments ; but these seem to point to mutable afflictions, such as are common in all accidents ; and there is a special prominence of Virgo and Scorpio. Aries and Leo are signs that often take to engineering, and so lay themselves open to accidents of this kind ; perhaps these signs have an affinity with steel ; perhaps Leo is common because when it is rising Aries is often on the meridian. Gemini-Sagittarius is well represented.

Cases

Mach 1—Male, born 8.10 a.m., 25.6.1891, Holt, Wilts. This is Case No. 1 in S.D., and shows heavy typical mutable afflictions ; Leo rises, with a malefic in Virgo—always a warning to avoid machines.

Mach 2—Male, born 7.29 a.m., 16.5.1900, 122° W., 48° N. Most of the fingers torn off in a piece of mill-machinery. Nothing in Virgo, but heavy Gemini-Sagittarius afflictions. The asc. is almost the same degree as that occupied by Mars in Mach 1.

Mach 3—Male, 12 p.m., 1.12.1900, Falkland Islands. At twenty-five lost his arm through falling into ship's machinery.

Mach 4—Child killed by being caught in farm-machinery, born 7.30 p.m., 17.10.1906, near London. I have not the reference for the source of this case, which has been published elsewhere unless my memory is mistaken.

A fifth case is given below. It is of interest that in these five we find Mars in Virgo in three, and in a fourth Saturn is in that sign.

Example No. 20

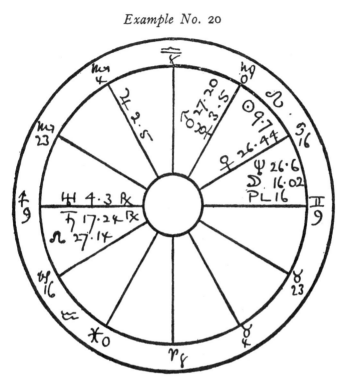

Man, born 4 p.m., August 1, 1899, Bath. He was killed (13.7.1916) when working a crane. He put his head through a gear-wheel, which started to revolve.

Circumstantial

A terribly afflicted map, there being three series of mutable afflictions, at the beginnings, middle, and ends of this cross. The Sun is natally fairly strong; but by direction it has to pass all these.

Tables

Mars and ascendant are in bad signs, and ☽, ♅, ♇ are in weak house-positions.

The stresses are mainly Uranian :   ⊙ ♅, ☽ ♅, ☿ ♅, ♄ ♇.

Directions

Asc. ☌ ♇ o-d, ♅ ☌ asc. ¼°.
♂ p. ☌ M.C.r.

§ 16. RAILWAY ACCIDENTS

IT is not easy to find many cases of these.

A case that is given in N.N. (No. 405) is that of a woman who was in a " dreadful " railway accident, so that her hair turned white. Six bodies are here in fixed signs, of which five are in a cross. They are Sun, Moon, Mercury, Uranus, and Pluto, the last from cusp 9th. Mars and Saturn are conjoined in Pisces in 6th. A bad map altogether. Venus is in the midst of minor bad aspects ; and perhaps this body rules the hair.

In A.Q., September 1930, a case (ref. RL 1) is given of a man who was cut to pieces at a railway crossing when motoring with friends after a convivial evening. The data are : Born 7.35 a.m., 11.3.1901, Paramatta, N.S.W. Killed 15.3.1930. Here there are six bodies in mutables, with heavy affliction. Uranus is opposed to Pluto and Sun-Mercury is in square to both. The Moon is square Mars.

RL 2—A lady born about 4 p.m., 2.5.1888, Cambridge. She and her husband were involved in the Lyons disaster of March 1924, the latter being killed. She was badly injured, chiefly in the foot. Some months later she died of cancer.

Earlier in life she had burnt her fingers in a laboratory with acid, causing permanent disfigurement.

This natus shows a close rising conjunction of Mars and Uranus—a very serious warning in any map. In itself this indicates dangerous experiences and the death of the partner. A more precise indication is the close opposition Jupiter-Pluto, cusps 3rd-9th. There is a rather wide, but effective, fixed " T," the Moon being opposite Saturn, with Sun-Mercury in square to both. Mars helio. is in 2° ♏, ☍ cusp 8th and forming a grand square with ☽, ♅, ♄.

Cancer is said (in E.P.A.) to be usually indicated by a Sun-Jupiter-Saturn complex ; and this we see here, since Saturn is in Leo (and in wide square to the Sun) and also in near trine to Jupiter. The Sun is also near to the quincunx to Mars and Uranus.

At the time of death Venus, ruler 1st and 8th, is conjoined with Neptune in the 8th by 1° ; and by ¼° we see that Mars and Uranus are opposed to her radical position. By 1° Pluto is square the ascendant.

A fourth case (RL 3) has a special interest. This is of a lady born at Moline, Illinois, 4.30 a.m., 6.7.1908. On 10.1.1927, she stepped from her husband's car to cross an electric railway-track, was caught by the foot in a hole left by workmen beneath a rail, and, unable to extricate herself, was deprived of both legs by the oncoming train. Her life was probably saved by her husband's promptitude in rushing her to hospital. She received heavy damages from the firm engaged on repairing the line.   Strong, pleasing personality ;   she surprised all by her fortitude and cheerfulness.

This map shows no less than 10 *squares and* 5 *oppositions,* and only 2 major good aspects.   Jupiter in 2nd shows the compensation received.   It is a peculiar map for loss of limbs, the afflictions, terrible as they are, being cardinal.   Almost all of them are forming. Uranus is certainly the major afflictor, and thus his rulership of railways is supported.

Now if we refer to page 121, "Spleen," we find there details of a German born the same day and with a nativity better only in that the Moon was past 8 ♄ and in close $*$ ♃ .

We do not often find horoscopes for the same day, and to compare them is very instructive, if sometimes rather baffling. [1]

In neither case does the heavy Cancer satellitium seem to have affected the character of the misfortune very explicitly, but each is distinctly Uranian.

§ 17.   POISON

DEATH by accidental poisoning is happily not very common ;   and in order to try to find a factor that is indicative of this sort of mischance I have used suicidal maps, and also one of murder—all involving the use of poison.

These unite in one very striking feature—in 10 cases used, Jupiter occupies Aquarius in no less than 6.   In

[1] See also V 7 and V 24.

2 more he is in square to bodies in that sign ; in another he is in the opposite sign Leo ; and thus in only one does he appear to have no connection with Aquarius at all. His relation with Aquarius in poison cases thus seems to be actual, if not invariable, whatever the reason may be.

The following cases show the degree-areas commonly affected :

SC 5	♄ 27 ♌	♂ 11 ♐
P 1	♅ 25 ♌	——
Suicide 4.	♃ 26 ♏	Asc. 10 ♐
5.	♄ 28 ♌	☿ 13 ♓
6.	♃ 26 ♌	☿ 12 ♐
7.	♅ 23 ♌	♂ 15 ♓
8.	♃ 28 ♒	☽ 16 ♊
N.N. 298	♂ 27 ♒	☉ 9 ♐ , asc. 16 ♐
450	♅ 27 ♉	☉ 12 ♓
525	♃ 24 ♒	——

Data for P 1 are given below. Suicide 4 and 5 are in S.D. Suicide 6, 7, and 8 are, respectively : sex not recorded, 11.41 p.m., 3.1.1861, 52½° N., 0° E., death 26.3.1902 ; male, 10 a.m., 12.7.1877, Geneva, died 30.6.1922 ; female, 2.30 p.m., 17.10.1867, Geneva, died 7.7.1922. All cases of poison.

Neptune is a common afflictor, and so too is Pluto, especially in relation to Mars.

I doubt if any hard-and-fast rules can be laid down for distinguishing suicide cases from accidental ones, and for distinguishing either or both of these classes from that of victims of murderous attacks. Perhaps the condition of the ruler and ascendant would be the most useful factor in this connection. But, even so, we get concurrences, as, for example, that Sagittarius has a high accident-ratio and also a marked suicidal propensity. These three classes would also, of course, often overlap. Suicides might have suffered both from accidents and from assaults, and so on.

P 1 is a case the source of which I have unfortunately not recorded, but it appears to be a birth at or near London, for about 3.46 p.m., May 7, 1878, and the note is, " Woman drank laudanum at about three and a half years, but recovered."

This case has resemblances to SC 5. Both have Venus in Aries ; in SC 5 she is opposed to Uranus, in P 1 she is conjunction Saturn and square Mars. In each Jupiter is in almost the same degree of Aquarius, in one in square, and in the other in trine, to Neptune. Neither map would be in danger of being mistaken for a map of self-destruction, but SC 5 has a notable resemblance to S.D. 6, which was for a birth only about a fortnight earlier and is itself something of a puzzle, since it contains numerous apparently good and strong aspects.

§ 18. EXPLOSIONS

THESE, like the foregoing, do not seem to be common, and I have only five cases.

N.N. 800 is that of a collier killed in a mine explosion.

There is a case, the source of which is, I think, M.A., though I have not kept a record, of a youth blown up in the *Bulwark*. Born December 17, 1894, asc. 28° ♋ .

This, of course, is not an accident, in the sense in which we have defined the term, unless the explosion could have been proved to be accidental and not due to enemy action. Furthermore, in such cases it is not easy to know exactly how any one individual met his end.

Thirdly, male, born 3.30 a.m., October 30, 1888, Bristol ; he was in a gas explosion and suffered shock.

Fourthly, the interesting case below.

Fifthly, a case given on page 109, A.Q., June, 1931. Boy, born 10.15 a.m., Pacific standard time, 12.1.1922, 123° 50′ W., 49° N. Blew himself up with charges used for blowing out the roots of trees. For full details see A.Q., but note erratum, as explained in the September issue, page 172. A most interesting case. Those who distrust the grand trine will ascribe the accident to that configuration between ☽, ♂ , and ♅ , whilst admitting that the child was fortunate enough to escape serious results from this and other adventures. Note Moon conjunction Pluto on cusp 5th ; the child's mishaps were mostly in play. This map was not included in the compilation of the tables, but it shows several weak elements, as ☿ and ♅ in unfavourable houses and ☽ and ♂ in bad signs.

These cases, for what so small a number may be worth, do not bear out the common belief that Uranus rules explosions. They have this common factor—that in all of them Neptune has an opposition. Uranus afflicts violently only in the colliery case (opposition asc.). Two cases have Moon at the beginning of Virgo, and a third has Mars there. In all five the Moon is in aspect with Mars—4 trines and 1 square.

Example No. 21

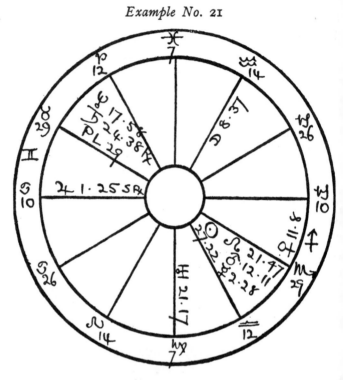

Male, born 8.50 p.m., October 20, 1882, Bath. When carrying out experiments with the inventor of a patent coffee-roaster, he burnt his face and hands severely through an explosion caused by his lighting a match when the gas was on.

The ☽ ♂ ♆ diathesis accounts for this accident, and would lead one to suspect a certain precipitancy in the native. The case nicely illustrates the Kennison reaction-points, for rpt. ♅ is exactly ☍ ♀, and rpt. ♆ exactly ☌ ☽. But the map is not a difficult one to interpret in any case. Those who believe that one can legitimately trace even details in the horoscope will explain that the Cancer ascendant signifies the domestic character of the coffee-roaster. The Sun in Libra and the Moon in Aquarius are certainly in character with the circumstances, which involved association.

☿, ♀, and ♂ are in bad signs.

§ 19. INJURIES FROM ANIMALS

THESE do not strictly come under the definition of accident, for there is no lack of intention in the dog's bite or the horse's kick. However, a short section on this subject may be of use, and certainly such cases are colloquially referred to as accidents.

The prime indication seems to be a Mars-Saturn-Jupiter complex. Example No. 8, on page 65, is a case in point ; here Mars is in a Jupiter sign and Jupiter is in trine to Saturn, the operative aspect being almost certainly Sun square Mars.

N.N. 63, " Bullfighter," shows Saturn rising in a sign of Mars and in aspect to Jupiter, whilst Moon square Saturn is the operative aspect.

AN 1—Girl, born about 4 p.m., 14.6.1923, Sydney, N.S.W. At two was kicked by a horse and was desperately ill. Mars is square Saturn but trine Jupiter, rising in a Mars sign. Lights square Uranus is the operative aspect.

AN 2—Lady, born 9.40 p.m., 28.11.1864, Walsall, Staffs. Severe dog-bite in summer of 1876. Mars afflicts Jupiter and Saturn and both lights are involved.

AN 3—Lady, born 8.40 p.m., 13.9.1889, Birmingham.

Bitten by a dog. Mars conj. Saturn and both trine Jupiter, which is square Sun.

See also CR 6, page 80, and William III, where an harmonious ♂ – ♃ – ♄ configuration is " broken " by ♅ ♆ ♌.

In a case of several bad dog-bites the two malefics are conjoined in Pisces, thus both coming under the Jupiter influence.

The question of the rulership of the different kinds of animals is a difficult one, and there seems very little agreement either in tradition or among modern writers. Gregarious animals probably come under Aquarius, at least in part, and there seems little doubt that horses come under the two Jovian signs, Jupiter and Neptune. Bulls, to mention a third species that sometimes is the source of serious injuries, would be automatically placed under Taurus, but N.N. 63 has nothing in that sign, and seems to respond to it chiefly through the opposite sign Scorpio. I know two other men who had narrow escapes from bulls—one had both lights in Scorpio square Saturn, and the other had severe Martian afflictions in cardinals : neither had anything in Taurus.

Two cases of stings from insects (severe) :

Wasps : female, born about 0.30 a.m., 18.6.1904, near London.

Bees : female, born 0.30 p.m., 20.5.1880, Boston, Mass.

In both cases there are afflictions in the radix between Uranus and the Sun, in both cases in Gemini. This sign appears, from these examples, to have affinity with the insect kingdom.

There is also W 2—a wasp-sting. This may be indicated by ♃ □ ♅ but more probably by ☿ ☌ ♂ ♊.

F 31 (thrown from horse) is a fine example of the ♂ - ♃ - ♄ complex, for these bodies, in this map, form a powerful grand trine, involving ♈ and ♐ .

I have no cases of snake-bites, anciently connected with the fixed star Fomalhaut in the beginning of the Fishes. Such, of course, are almost as rare in England nowadays as they are in Ireland, but there should be plenty of cases among Anglo-Indians, as well as natives of the tropics.

§ 20. LOCALISATION

THIS subject alone might occupy the attention of years of close study. However, it seems that upon the whole the traditional teachings regarding astro-physiology are correct. In this section I have endeavoured to classify a number of cases already given, according to the parts of the body affected. This may serve as a basis for future detailed research, and some of the results of even this elementary examination of the subject may be useful.

The Head

Cases are : Exx. Nos. 11, 13, 18.

F 14, 17, 33.

N.N. 853, 976.

V 4.

These nine cases show no special Aries incidence ; there is, therefore, no support for the traditional connection between this sign and the head.

But the ascendant is plainly significant in this relation. Taking the above cases in order, we find :

Ex. 11   ♅ rising ☐ ruler 1st
    13   ♃   ,,   ☐ ♄ ♀ , △ lord 1st
    18   ♃   ,,   ☍ ♄ ☐ ♇.
F 14   ♄   ,,   ♂ ♇ ☐ ☉ ☿
F 17   Asc. ☐ ♄
F 33   Ruler 1st ☿ , ☐ ♂
N.N. 853 ♅ rising
    976   ♇   ,,   (curious   case,   nothing
            cardinal)
V 4   ♄ setting (he is 8° from cusp 7th, but
            time is approximate ; he may be
            asc.)

Mars afflictions are, respectively :

    1.   ☐ ♄
    2.   ☍ ☽
    3.   nil
    4.   ☍ ♀ ☐ ♃
    5.   ☐ ☉ ☿
    6.   ☐ ☿ ♀
    7.   ♂ ☉ ☿
    8.   ☍ ☉
    9.   ☐ ♅

It is evident from this that Mars is often heavily afflicted in these cases.

So, too, is Mercury.

Mars tends also to be near the end of signs. In these 9 cases his average degree = 24°.

N.N. 976 is the only case in which the ascendant is not afflicted either by Saturn or by Uranus. This affliction is perhaps the chief index.

Areas that appear marked are : About 22° cardinals and the end of the fixed signs (21°–27°).

The Face

   Exx. Nos. 6, 10, 14, 21.
   B 6.
   BL 19.
   SC 2.
   N.N. 832.

These show the asc. afflicted by Saturn, or, less often, by Mars, Jupiter, or Uranus.   Thus :

Ex.	6	♄ ☌ asc.	
	10	♃ ☉ ☌ asc., ☍ ♂	
	14	♄ ☍ asc.	
	21	♄ ∠ asc.	
SC	2	♄ (debilitated) △ asc.	
BL	19	♅ ☌ asc.	
N.N.	832	♅ ☌ asc.	

We may also here note the reappearance of the area 22° cardinals (especially ♈ ♎), and this is often under Venus or Saturn influence.   Thus :

Ex.	6	♀ 22° ♎	
	14	♄ 22° ♈	
	21	☉ 27° ♎	
SC	12	♄ 20° ♈	
B.	19	☉ 23° ♈	
N.N.	832	♆ 25° ♈	

I have noticed the same areas in facial disfigurement by eczema. In fact, this disease was very troublesome in a case almost identical with Ex. 6. The fixed-sign area (around 23°) also occurs in facial disfigurement.

Where the appearance is disfigured, as distinct from cranial injury only, one might expect a severe Venus affliction, since the personal beauty is affected. This seems, in fact, to be the case. In Ex. 10 Venus is in good aspect with Saturn, Uranus, and Neptune, but even the benefic aspects of three malefics is not likely to lend charm to the appearance.

A characteristic case is Misc. 7 (lady, born in New York City, about midnight, 30/31.12.1872). She fell owing to faintness, and hit her face on a chair. Mars rises in 19½ ♎, 8 ♅ 23° ♈, □ ☽ 24° ♑, ♄ 22° ♑. This illustrates the cardinal area very forcefully. ♀ 21° ♒ touches the fixed area.

The Jaw

BL 6 shows both the areas above mentioned— ♀ 23° ♑, ♅ 23° ♒, ♄ is 8 ascendant.

I should be inclined to place the jaw, a powerful muscle much used, at least in primitive times, in battle, under ♂, which in this case is □ ♄.

♂ ♐ shows danger from vehicles.

Collar-bone

Three cases illustrate broken collar-bones:

W 2, F 7, F 26.

In these we see ☽ 8 ♅, ☽ □ ♄, ☽ 8 ♄; two show a combination of ♊ and ♋.

Breast

Case : B 7. I am inclined to place this organ under Venus-Libra rather than under Moon-Cancer, as is traditionally supposed. Here Venus-Libra is involved, but so also are the Moon and Cancer. I found my belief chiefly upon certain cases of amputation, due to disease.

The Arms

These may be placed for the chief part under Virgo, with an occasional action in Pisces, by polarity. Sometimes Mercury bears the affliction, and Gemini-Sagittarius are often involved.

Cases are :

SC 3   Flesh taken off the left arm by scalding. ☉ ♓ ∠ ♅.

B 7   Arms burnt.   ☉ ♍ □ ♅.

B 8   Arms burnt.   ♂ ♄ rising in ♓.

Mach 1   Arm torn off.   ♄ ♍ ☍ ♃ ♓.

Mach 3   Lost arm.   ♂ ♍ □ ☉ ♐.

Misc 9   Male, 12.30 p.m., 7.12.1901, Manchester. Broke left arm.   ☉ ♂ ♅ ♐, ☿ ♐ □ asc. ♓.

V 1   Right arm broken.   ♂ ♓.

F 3   Fractured arm.   5° ♍ asc. ☍ ♅.

F 12   Left arm fractured.   □ ♂ asc. in ♐.

N.N. 157 Fractured arm.   ☽ ♍ ☍ ♅ ♓ ; ♄ ♓.

Hands

Gemini-Virgo afflictions seem common, and there is

usually a contact between Mercury and Mars, though not always a bad one.

W 2 Badly cut hands with broken bottle. ☿ ☌ ♂ ♊.
B 5 Burnt skin off the right hand. ☿ ♊ ⚹ ♂ ♈.
BL 5 Back of hand badly knocked. ☿ ☉ ♂ rising in ♍ □ ♃ ♆ PL in ♊.

Fingers

These seem to come under the positive mutables.

Ex. 8 Fingers broken. ☉ ♊ □ ♂.
W 3 Cut off a finger. ♄ ♊.
Mach 2 Fingers torn off. ☽ ☌ ♅ ♐ ☍ PL.
CR 6 Finger cut when mowing. ☉ ♐, ♂ ♍ ☍ ☽ ♓.
Misc 3 Male, 4.55 p.m., 12.12.1893, New York City. Two broken fingers, one through a fall in skating, and one in playful wrestling ; right finger seriously cut with glass ; bridge of nose smashed when skating, Christmas 1921. ☉ ♐ ☍ ♆ ; for nose, see ♏ afflictions.

The Spine

Some of the cases show striking resemblances.

F 5 ☉ 9 ♍ □ ♄ 6 ♐ ; ♂ 29 ♊.
F 7 ☉ ☿ ♆ ☍ ♂ 5 ♐ ; asc. 29 ♍.
F 8 ♂ 3 ♐ ; ♄ 1 ♋.
F 27 cusp 12th 5 ♐ ; ♂ 2 ♋.

As will be seen above, two areas seem to be involved.

The Pelvis

   Cases are : F 6, BL 18.

   These resemble the spine cases in the occurrence of positions at the beginnings of the mutables.

$$F \; 6 \quad \odot \; 3 \; \text{⋇} \; \square \; \mars \; 5 \; \text{♐}.$$
$$BL \; 18 \quad \jupiter \; 4 \; \text{⋇} \; 8 \; \uranus.$$

Spleen

   Two cases :

   BL 17.

   Misc 2 : Male, 5 a.m., 5.9.1915, Scranton, Pa. Lost spleen by reason of an accident.

   Cancer satellitia in both cases.

Bladder

   See Ex. No. 8 ♅ 12 ♏, 8 cusp 8th is probably responsible.

   Curiously, a case of death as a result of an operation on the bladder (male, 12 p.m., 8.5.1836, Lancs) also shows ♅ on the cusp of the 2nd.   ♄ in 1° ♏ △ ☽ ♅ but □ ♆.

Liver

   Exx. 9 and 17.

   These show very similar afflictions involving the ends of Virgo-Pisces. This area is certainly related to the liver.

Legs

   Fractured legs are most commonly represented by bad aspects in mutables and by Jupiter afflictions.

Often Mars afflicts this planet, and very commonly Mars is in a Jovian sign or Jupiter in a Martian. Jupiter seems also often to be in Leo. There are less often Jupiter-Saturn afflictions, and occasionally Saturn and Capricorn are concerned, rather than Jupiter and Sagittarius, even though the particulars of the accident do not mention the knee.

An important area is 10° ♈ (less often ♋, ♎ or ♑).

Cases

F	6	Right leg removed. ♃ ♏ ☍ ♆, etc.
V	1	Thigh broken. ♂ ♓, ♀ 10 ♈, ♃ ♌.
V	24	Right leg amputated. ♃ ☌ ♂ ♈.
Ex	19	Thigh burnt. ♃ 9° ♈.
RL	3	Legs cut off. ♄ 10° ♈, ♃ ♌.
SC	6	Scalded legs. ♃ ♌, ♂ 10° ♈.
SC	10	Scalded legs. ☽ 13 ♈, ♃ 19 ♈, ♄ 29 ♈.
V	7	Leg broken. ♃ ☌ ♂ ♈, cp. V 24.
V	15	Broke leg. ♃ ☌ ♂, ☽ 11° ♑.
BL	2	Left leg lost. ♃ ☌ ♂.
BL	4	Left leg lost. ♃ ♏, ☉ ⚹ □ ♅.
BL	7	Smashed leg. ♃ ♌ □ ♄, ☿ 11° ♎.
BL	9	Both legs fractured. ♂ 8° ♎ □ ♄.
BL	19	Leg amputated. ♃ 13° ♑ ☌ ♄ ; ☿ □ ♆ (sepsis).
F	1	Leg broken. ♃ ♐ ☍ ♅, ♂ 7° ♋ □ ♆.
F	2	Leg broken. ♃ ☍ ☿ ♄.
F	15	Legs broken surgically. ♃ ⚼ ♂, ♊ ♐ afflictions, ♃ 7° ♎.

Knee

BL 3 Knee-cap smashed. Apparently ☽ ♐ 8 ♃
        ♊, ♅ □ ☽ o-d at time.

F 9 Water on knee.   ♂ 9° ♑.

The 10° cardinals area seems also to apply here.

Feet

CR 6 Foot broken by horse.   ☽ ♓ 8 ♂.

F 12 Cut foot.   ♇ □ ♅ in 8th, also ♐ afflictions.

CR 4 Foot crushed.   ☉ ♐ 8 ♄.

W 4 Cut foot.   ♃ ♓ 8 ♇, □ ☿.

B 4 Foot burnt.   ♃ ♓.

F 13 Injuries to foot.   ♄ ♊ □ ♇.

Miscellaneous

A few odd cases follow. These may be of use for comparison.

Ankle	V 6
Eye	BL 1
Hair	N.N. 405
Kidney	BL 16
Nose	Misc 3, above
Teeth	The same
Tongue	Ex 14